URINARY TRACT INFECTION

Other titles in the *New Clinical Applications* Series:

Dermatology (Series Editor Dr J. L. Verbov)

Cardiology (Series Editor Dr D. Longmore)

Rheumatology (Series Editors Dr J. J. Calabro† and Dr W. Carson Dick)

Nephrology (Series Editor Dr G. R. D. Catto)

NEW CLINICAL APPLICATIONS NEPHROLOGY

URINARY TRACT INFECTION

Editor

G. R. D. CATTO

MD, DSc, FRCP, FRCP (Lond., Edin. and Glasg.)

Professor of Medicine
University of Aberdeen
UK

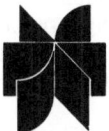

KLUWER ACADEMIC PUBLISHERS
DORDRECHT / BOSTON / LONDON

Distributors

for the United States and Canada: Kluwer Academic Publishers, PO Box 358,
Accord Station, Hingham, MA 02018–0358, USA
for all other countries: Kluwer Academic Publishers Group, Distribution
Center, PO Box 322, 3300 AH Dordrecht, The Netherlands

British Library Cataloguing in Publication Data

Urinary tract infection.
  1. Man. Urinary tract. Diseases
  I. Catto, Graeme R. D. (Graeme Robertson Dawson), *1945–*   II. Series
  616.6

Library of Congress Cataloging in Publication Data

Urinary tract infection.

  (New clinical applications. Nephrology)
  Includes bibliographies and index.
  1. Urinary tract infections.   I. Catto, Graeme R. D.
II. Series.   [DNLM: 1. Urinary Tract Infections.
WJ 151 U7595]
RC901.8.U748   1988   616.6   89–2836
ISBN-13: 978-94-010-6871-0   e-ISBN-13: 978-94-009-0853-6
DOI: 10.1007/978-94-009-0853-6

Copyright

Published in the United Kingdom by Kluwer Academic Publishers,
PO Box 55, Lancaster, UK.

Kluwer Academic Publishers BV incorporates the publishing programmes of
D. Reidel, Martinus Nijhoff, Dr W. Junk and MTP Press.

CONTENTS

LIST OF AUTHORS

C. E. Daman Willems
  Renal Unit
  Hospital for Sick Children
  Great Ormond Street
  London, WC1N 3JN
  UK

R. Maskell
  Wessex Renal Unit and Public
    Health Laboratory
  St Mary's Hospital
  East Wing, Milton Road
  Portsmouth, PO3 6AQ
  UK

S. McClinton
  Department of Urology
  Ward 44, Aberdeen Royal
    Infirmary
  Foresterhill
  Aberdeen, AB9 2ZB
  UK

L. E. F. Moffat
  Department of Urology
  Ward 44, Aberdeen Royal
    Infirmary
  Foresterhill
  Aberdeen, AB9 2ZB
  UK

D. J. Propper
  Department of Medicine and
    Therapeutics
  Polwarth Building
  Foresterhill
  Aberdeen, AB9 2ZD
  UK

J. M. Smellie
  Department of Paediatrics
  University College Hospital
  Gower Street
  London, WC1E 6AU
  UK

SERIES EDITOR'S FOREWORD

Urinary tract infection remains one of the most common reasons for an individual seeking medical advice. Although the associated morbidity varies widely in adults, such infections are less common but may constitute severe, life-threatening illness in children and in the elderly. Diagnostic tests and treatment have been rationalized in recent years but many practising doctors still have difficulty in appreciating the patho-physiological principles involved.

Particular difficulty is often experienced when treating patients with recurrent urinary tract infections, covert bacteriuria, vesico-ureteric reflux, elderly patients and those with indwelling catheters. These topics are fully discussed in this volume. Each chapter has been written by a recognized expert and practical aspects of patient management have been emphasized. The information presented in this volume should prove of interest not only to nephrologists but to all practising clinicians.

ABOUT THE EDITOR

Professor Graeme R. D. Catto is Professor in Medicine and Therapeutics at the University of Aberdeen and Honorary Consultant Physician/Nephrologist to the Grampian Health Board. His current interest in transplant immunology was stimulated as a Harkness Fellow at Harvard Medical School and the Peter Bent Brighton Hospital, Boston, USA. He is a member of many medical societies including the Association of Physicians of Great Britain and Ireland, the Renal Association and the Transplantation Society. He has published widely on transplant and reproductive immunology, calcium metabolism and general nephrology.

1

RECURRENT URINARY TRACT INFECTIONS INCLUDING COVERT BACTERIURIA

R. MASKELL

INTRODUCTION

During the past thirty years there have been many important changes in the diagnosis and management of urinary tract infection (UTI), and research undertaken during this period has led to a better understanding of the significance of bacteriuria. The great upsurge of interest in the subject in the sixties and seventies, in response to the work of Kass, has been followed by the workload and financial pressures of the eighties. Decisions must constantly be made, by clinicians and by laboratories, about the appropriate use of resources in the diagnosis and management of UTI. It is useful, therefore, to survey the current state of knowledge in the field and to endeavour to lay down some guidelines for laboratory and clinical work. Aspects which will be considered in this review will include a concept of UTI which takes account of infection anywhere in the urinary tract or its adjacent structures rather than, as has been customary, confining attention to the kidneys and bladder only; the changes in laboratory methods and diagnosis which have resulted from this concept; the clinical significance of UTI, the management of symptoms, and ways in which the small minority of bacteriuric patients who are at risk from serious consequences may be identified; antibacterial agents and management protocols and, finally, the problem of covert bacteriuria.

INFECTIONS OF THE URINARY TRACT AND ADJACENT STRUCTURES

Significant bacteriuria

The concept of 'significant bacteriuria' originated from the work of Kass[1,2] who validated the midstream specimen (MSU) as a means of diagnosing bladder bacteriuria. This was soon acccepted as synonymous with urinary tract infection – a proposition which, almost from the outset, was shown to be unsatisfactory but which, largely for simplicity of clinical and laboratory diagnosis, has persisted. The definition of 'significant bacteriuria', as enunciated by Kass from culture of first early morning MSU specimens from symptom-free women, has been generally accepted as the presence of at least 100 000 organisms of a recognized aerobic urinary pathogen, usually in pure culture, per ml of a fresh carefully-collected MSU – the finding preferably confirmed in a repeat specimen. The limitations of this definition in the clinical context are obvious, but it is only in very recent years that attention has been paid to these limitations and efforts have been made to provide more accurate diagnosis.

The most obvious fallacies in the concept of 'significant bacteriuria' relate to bacterial count and bacterial species. A high count is dependent upon incubation of organisms in the bladder urine for a sufficient length of time; the possibility of lower counts, either due to the presence of bacteria in tissues such as the kidney or prostate, whence they may be shed into the urine in small numbers, or to the constant dilution of the bacterial count in the bladder that occurs in patients with severe frequency and thirst, is ignored. Secondly, it has been accepted too readily that only the aerobic organisms, which can survive in the relatively high oxygen tension of bladder urine and are easily detected by overnight aerobic culture, cause urinary tract infection.

The criterion of 'significant bacteriuria' with an aerobic pathogen provides no explanation for the symptoms of about one-half of the women and two-thirds of the men who present with urinary symptoms – the symptoms in these patients usually being clinically indistinguishable from those with 'significant bacteriuria'. It also leaves much pyuria unexplained. The validity of low counts of aerobic organisms was addressed many years ago, and there was evidence, both from suprapubic aspiration (SPA)[3] and catheterization[4], that

2

organisms were often present in the bladder urine in counts of fewer than 10^5/ml. The recent work of Stamm and his colleagues[5] has again drawn attention to this fact. However, even when low counts have been accepted as significant[6] and more attention paid to purity than to count (it is impossible for a urine specimen to be contaminated with a single bacterial species, the sites from which contamination may occur all having a mixed commensal flora), the symptoms of many patients and much pyuria have remained unexplained.

In recent years, progress has been made towards a better understanding of urinary symptoms by enlarging the concept of UTI to include the whole urinary tract, above and below the bladder, and its adjacent structures, and by considering the possibility that, in some sites and under some particular circumstances, organisms other than the recognized aerobic pathogens may be responsible for infection. It seems reasonable to suppose that microaerophilic organisms which cannot survive in the oxygen tension of bladder urine could multiply and cause infection in the prostate or paraurethral tissues of women, or in scarred bladder or kidney tissue. There is now a large body of evidence that such organisms can be isolated from the urine of patients with prostatitis, urethral syndrome, chronic pyelonephritic scarring, and chronic or 'interstitial' cystitis. This evidence was reviewed[7] in 1986 and more recent studies have confirmed the findings[8,9]. The changes in laboratory diagnostic methods necessitated by these new considerations of bacterial counts and urinary pathogens are discussed below.

Localization of infection within the urinary tract

One of the major clinical problems in the diagnosis and management of UTI is the difficulty of determining the site of infection within the urinary tract. With the exception of the classical symptoms and signs of acute pyelonephritis it is not possible to determine the site of infection by clinical means, and there has been disappointingly little progress in the development of laboratory tests for this purpose. Clinical diagnosis is bedevilled by the problem of referred pain – for example from the bladder or urethra to the loin – and by the important phenomenon of apparently asymptomatic infection. Culture of urine specimens

3

obtained by ureteric catheterization under general anaesthesia remains the only definitive way of proving kidney infection; for obvious reasons, this is not a procedure which is often undertaken. Laboratory tests, such as the detection of antibody-coated bacteria or P-fimbriated bacteria in the urine, have not proved definitive and are not in general use. Bladder infection can be confirmed by SPA, which is now often undertaken in babies but seldom in adults, and prostatic infection may be detected by collection of urine after prostatic massage. However, in general clinical practice, the diagnosis of UTI depends upon microscopy and culture of an MSU, and it is on the interpretation of the findings of this investigation that the majority of clinicians rely.

CHANGES IN LABORATORY DIAGNOSTIC METHODS

It is regrettable that the widespread acceptance of Kass' numerical criteria of significance led rapidly to a more rigid unthinking approach to urine microbiology than had been practised previously. In many laboratories the interpretation of urine cultures was delegated to laboratory scientific workers, often quite junior and usually without the clinical insight required for such interpretation. Few had actually read Kass' papers or were aware of the limitations of the numerical criterion which Kass himself acknowledged. The possibility of infection of tissues below the bladder, and the likelihood of lower bacterial counts from infections in that situation, were ignored. The fact that bacteriuria can be significant in the absence of pyuria was used, in some laboratories, as a reason for dispensing with urine microscopy as a routine procedure; the obvious fact that pyuria may be very important in the apparent absence of bacteriuria was forgotten. During the years that these new practices were developing – years of the great increase in laboratory workload and the consequent financial pressures – evidence of the significance of low bacterial counts, of apparently 'sterile' pyuria, and of the pathogenicity of organisms other than aerobes in parts of the urinary tract and its adjacent structures was accumulating. As clinicians begin to accept this new evidence and to require more extensive and accurate work from laboratories, the latter are faced with the difficulty of reversing the trend away from interpretation by rules of thumb and moving towards protocols which require greater

4

medical input and consideration of the findings in each urine specimen on its merits. Factors which must now be taken into account include the age and sex of the patient, the type of specimen (for example MSU or indwelling catheter specimen), pyuria, bacterial count and purity of growth, and relevant clinical factors including antibacterial treatment. This approach has two major advantages – it is more likely to provide the correct result for each individual patient and thus to prompt appropriate clinical management, and it results in wiser use of antibacterial agents, with all the advantages to individual patients and the community in general which are consequent on this. Both these considerations will be discussed later.

Adopting this new approach, however, is not easy at a time when financial and workload pressures are increasing and the advent of serious new infections threatens to take up an ever greater proportion of laboratory resources. To those who question the justification for giving the time, thought and some additional resources to undertaking accurate and useful laboratory work in the field of UTI, it is salutary to pose two other questions. Is the money spent on examining large numbers of urine specimens using rules of thumb for interpretation, and providing results which may be inaccurate, unhelpful, often irrelevant and sometimes harmful, wasted? In view of the very large number of patients who suffer from urinary symptoms, is it not wiser to spend a little extra on accurate laboratory diagnosis than to incur the considerable expense of repeated antibacterial treatment and investigations which are often unnecessary and sometimes harmful?

Laboratory procedures

Without entering into too many technicalities, the major changes in laboratory procedures which enlarge the diagnostic potential of urine microscopy and culture are:

1. Incubation of cultures in an atmosphere containing 7–10% CO_2. This technique is now widely used for incubation of cultures from other diagnostic specimens, such as swabs and blood cultures; it is equally necessary for urine cultures.

2. Incubation for 48 h of cultures from patients with symptoms,

pyuria, or organisms seen on microscopy which are unexplained by overnight culture. 48 h incubation will reveal the presence of the majority of fastidious organisms which are present in the urine.

3. Use of culture media additional to the primary isolation medium for examination of specimens from patients with symptoms or pyuria in whom the above procedures have yielded negative results. This will only be required for a small minority of specimens. It can also usefully be employed in the first instance for specimens from patients with particular clinical syndromes in which fastidious organisms requiring these additional media have been shown to be important, e.g. 'interstitial cystitis', prostatitis, post-prostatectomy infection, epididymo-orchitis, and infection in patients undergoing pelvic radiotherapy.

Interpretation and reporting of urine cultures

If the correct interpretation of urine microscopy and culture is to be made, every specimen must be considered 'on its merits'. The factors which must be taken into account have already been listed; if the report is to be intelligible and helpful to the requesting clinician, it must be factual and carry an interpretation comment if necessary. Terms such as 'no significant growth', which are often applied at the bench by non-medical laboratory staff, should not be used. They usually indicate a mechanical approach to interpretation and ignore the clinical context. For example, a low count of a Gram-negative organism may be of considerable significance in an adult male with prostatitis and certainly requires sensitivity tests, whereas a high count of such an organism in an elderly woman with an indwelling catheter when she is well and symptom free is not significant; sensitivity testing of the isolate will almost certainly prompt ill-advised antibacterial treatment and is contraindicated. The former, however, will often be reported as 'no significant growth' whereas the latter is likely to be reported as significant. There are many other such examples.

Therefore, in reporting urine cultures, the identity and count of the isolates should be stated (obvious contaminants, such as a mixed growth of urethral commensals may be recorded as 'mixed Gram-positive organisms') and a decision as to the significance of the isolates should be made by medical staff or by experienced scientific staff who have been trained appropriately. In the latter case, it should always remain open to medical staff to reconsider the interpretation put on the findings if necessary. It follows, of course, that this approach to correct diagnosis depends upon the accuracy and completeness of the request form that accompanies the specimen. In my experience, the relevant information required on such forms is only obtained if they are written by the doctor who makes the decision to request the investigation. I do not share the increasingly prevalent view that such forms may appropriately be written by nurses – still less by clerical staff. Restriction of laboratory requests for urine culture to those accompanied by a form actually written by a doctor will do more to save unnecessary, and often harmful, work than any other single effort in this direction.

Automated and screening procedures

In an attempt to solve the problem of increasing laboratory workloads in this field, many such procedures have been developed. The use of such techniques approaches the problem from the opposite direction from the one outlined above – instead of attempting to restrict the requests to appropriate and well-documented specimens, it presupposes that the number of specimens will continue to rise unchecked, and that ways must be found in the laboratory either to examine them rapidly using minimum labour or, by screening techniques, to select those which merit microscopy and culture and to discard the rest.

At the time of writing, there are many reasons why this approach should be rejected:

1. The published data show that the automated procedures at present available are insufficiently sensitive and specific to detect all significant infections (which, of course, include significant low bacterial counts)[10].

2. There are no published data on the detection of fastidious urinary pathogens by such methods.

3. Screening devices for selection of specimens for microscopy and culture, such as the various chemical dip sticks which are available, are insufficiently sensitive and specific[11], and their use does not result in an appreciable saving in time or money.

4. Any laboratory protocol which results in the acceptance of unlimited numbers of specimens, and the discarding of some of them unexamined, inevitably leads to poor liaison between clinician and laboratory in the diagnosis of UTI. It leads to increased use of antibacterial agents for treatment of symptoms without any attempt at laboratory diagnosis, with all the consequent disadvantages to patient and community in terms of side effects and resistant organisms, and loses the opportunity to educate clinicians in the appropriate use of the laboratory.

Restriction of laboratory workload by elimination of unnecessary specimens and laboratory procedures

This can be achieved in the following ways:

1. Insistence that, with a few agreed and necessary exceptions, all specimens should be accompanied by a request form written by a doctor.

2. Bacteriuria screening programmes, for example of pregnant women, should be discontinued if audit shows that communications are poor and the results are not acted on effectively.

3. Submission of specimens from patients with indwelling catheters at times when they are well should be discouraged. Sensitivity testing of isolates from such specimens should only be undertaken if the request form states specifically that the patient is unwell, feverish or confused.

4. Submission of 'routine' specimens from departments where specimen collection techniques are poor (e.g. bag specimens from babies) should be discouraged. Good specimens can be obtained from babies if the requesting doctor takes an interest in the method of specimen collection and transport.

5. 'Stix' testing of all urine specimens in the laboratory is unnecessary, wasteful and often inaccurate. If proteinuria testing is either requested or considered appropriate in the laboratory, an accurate test, such as the sulphosalicylic acid test, should be employed. Screening 'stix' tests are easily undertaken in clinical areas, and laboratory confirmation of positive tests may be requested.

6. Centrifugation of urine for microscopy is unnecessary, inaccurate and more time consuming than inverted microscopy of uncentrifuged urine.

7. A single primary isolation medium is sufficient for the great majority of urine specimens. The use of two or more media can be helpful if a multipoint inoculation technique is used, but the time and expertise required to interpret the findings of such techniques correctly is not always available. Direct plating methods need only one effective primary medium, for example CLED agar; the use of additional media is time consuming and expensive.

8. Full biochemical identification of all Gram-negative isolates is expensive and unnecessary except in the rare clinical circumstances of outbreaks of cross-infection, associated septicaemia, or isolation of very resistant (e.g. gentamicin-resistant) organisms. After brief screening tests to identify *Pseudomonas* spp, *Proteus* spp. and *Salmonella* spp., the remainder may be reported as 'coliform'. Any laboratory which finds it necessary to fully identify many Gram-negative urinary isolates for any of the reasons given above should suspect that there is something seriously wrong, either with instrumentation procedures or the use of broad-spectrum antibacterials, in its area. In our laboratory, we have occasion to identify only about 20 Gram-negative urinary isolates for all the above reasons each year.

9. Abbreviated methods for identification and reporting of Gram-positive urinary isolates, for example the use of novobiocin resistance for identification of *Staphylococcus saprophyticus*, have been validated and may be used in routine laboratory practice.

10. The culture of urine specimens for *Mycobacterium* spp. is rarely indicated. The presence of fastidious organisms as an explanation

for pyuria should first be sought by culture on appropriate media and prolonged incubation in 7–10% CO_2.

CLINICAL SIGNIFICANCE OF BACTERIURIA

There are three principal considerations in determining the significance of bacteriuria:

1. Is it giving rise to urinary symptoms with/without systemic upset?

2. Is it associated with, or the cause of, inflammatory changes in the kidneys, bladder, prostate or paraurethral tissues of women?

3. Is it associated with, or the cause of, calculi in the kidneys, bladder or prostate?

Urinary symptoms with/without systemic upset

Symptoms related to micturition – frequency, dysuria, nocturia, hae-maturia, pain, perineal discomfort, dyspareunia, urge incontinence or post-micturition dribble – may result from infection anywhere in the urinary tract and its adjacent structures. In addition, pain may be referred from the site of infection to other parts of the urinary tract. It is difficult to be dogmatic about the frequency with which systemic upset of any kind accompanies bacterial infection of the urinary tract – for example, the body temperature of women with cystitis is seldom recorded – but certain clinical syndromes in which systemic upset occurs are well recognized. The loin pain, fever, and rigors of acute pyelonephritis are characteristic, and many men with prostatitis are feverish and have evidence, such as rigors, of bacteraemia. Elderly patients often become acutely confused as a result of bac-teriuria and babies may be non-specifically unwell.

Until recently, as already mentioned, no infective cause was found for the urinary symptoms of one-half of the women and two-thirds of the men who present to their doctors, and many non-infective causes have been proposed. Failure to prove a definitive cause has often resulted, and regrettably still often results, in a variety of psychological diagnoses, including sex-related neurosis and general personality disorders. If the traditional concept of urinary tract infection is extended to include the urethra and related structures below the bladder, and if a thorough bacteriological search is made for a possible pathogen, the percentage of patients in whom an infective diagnosis can be made increases dramatically. Apart from those due to infection with aerobic or fastidious bacteria, it is likely that some symptoms may be associated with chlamydial cervicitis or urethritis[5], although it has been shown that women with proven chlamydial infection may deny any urinary symptoms, even on direct questioning[12]. Excretion of viruses in the urine during the course of viral infections may give rise to urinary symptoms, although few studies of viruria have been undertaken. It is almost certainly the cause of the transient micturition symptoms of which children sometimes complain at times when urine microscopy and culture are completely negative. Interestingly, there is one group of patients with symptoms in whom no cause has yet been demonstrated – boys up to the age of puberty. Bacterial urinary infection is not as uncommon in this population as is often believed – we found a ratio of 1:4 of symptomatic urinary infections in boys and girls from 2–12 years of age[13] – but, although many show positive urine microscopy and culture, an appreciable number of others (approximately 8–10 per week in our laboratory, which serves a population of over half a million people) yield completely negative results.

Chronic inflammatory changes in the urinary tract and related structures

Persistent or recurrent UTI or, it is believed, a single attack of UTI in some young children can give rise to inflammatory changes which, under certain circumstances, may become established and chronic.

Figure 1.1 shows, in diagrammatic fashion, the sites in the urinary tract where such infections occur. Chronic inflammation of the kidney and upper urinary tract is comparatively rare and presents a greater threat to life and health than infections of the bladder and below.

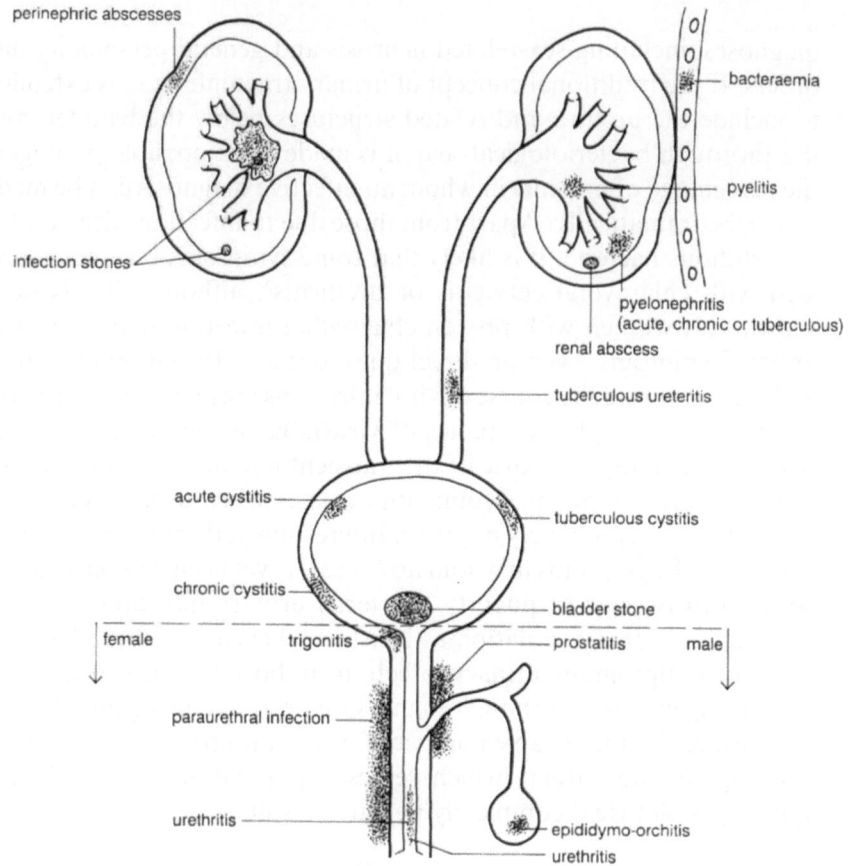

FIGURE 1.1   Diagrammatic representation of infective diseases of the urinary tract and adjacent structures. All conditions, with the exception of those below the bladder, may occur in either sex

Renal and perinephric infection

Blood-borne infection of the kidney is rare, but it may occur in staphylococcal or fungal septicaemia, resulting in multiple abscess formation. The majority of renal infections arise by the ascending route and the commonest predisposing cause is vesico-ureteric (v–u) reflux, either primary or secondary.

Primary v–u reflux will be considered in Chapter 2. It is principally a condition of children and seldom persists into adult life. Renal infection and chronic inflammation (chronic atrophic pyelonephritic scarring), therefore, begin in childhood, usually before the age of 5 years, but may extend and progress into adult life if left unchecked. If extensive and bilateral, infection may result in renal failure; even if it is unilateral, the secondary changes in the renal parenchyma, whether due to secondary glomerulonephritis or to hypertension, may also lead to loss of renal function.

Secondary v–u reflux may also occur in children or adults. It is possible that it is sometimes due to oedema and inflammation around the ureteric orifices resulting from persistent or recurrent bladder infection; it may also be acquired as a result of back pressure from bladder outlet obstruction due to bladder stones, posterior urethral valves, severe prostatic hypertrophy or urethral stricture. In conditions when bladder emptying is impaired as a result of neurological defect – neuropathic bladder – passive reflux may also occur; the likelihood of this is reduced in the low-pressure systems of ileal bladders and urostomies.

Bacteraemia may occur in the acute inflammatory stage of acute pyelonephritis. When infection is chronic, extension of infection to the perinephric space and the bloodstream usually occurs only if an element of obstruction is added. Characteristically, this occurs in the presence of infection stones which have grown to obstruct the collecting system. This condition will be considered later.

Bladder infection

It is likely that the majority of attacks of acute cystitis do not result in chronic inflammatory change in the bladder wall. They are due to multiplication in the urine of bacteria which reach the bladder by the ascending route. They respond rapidly to appropriate antibacterial therapy and there is evidence from electron microscopy studies that the bladder epithelium does not undergo structural damage[14] (Figure 1.2a). The situation is different, however, in patients who develop persistent or relapsing cystitis (Figure 1.2b). Disruption of the epithelium and of the protective mucin layer which provides the natural defence against bacterial invasion of the bladder allows organisms to

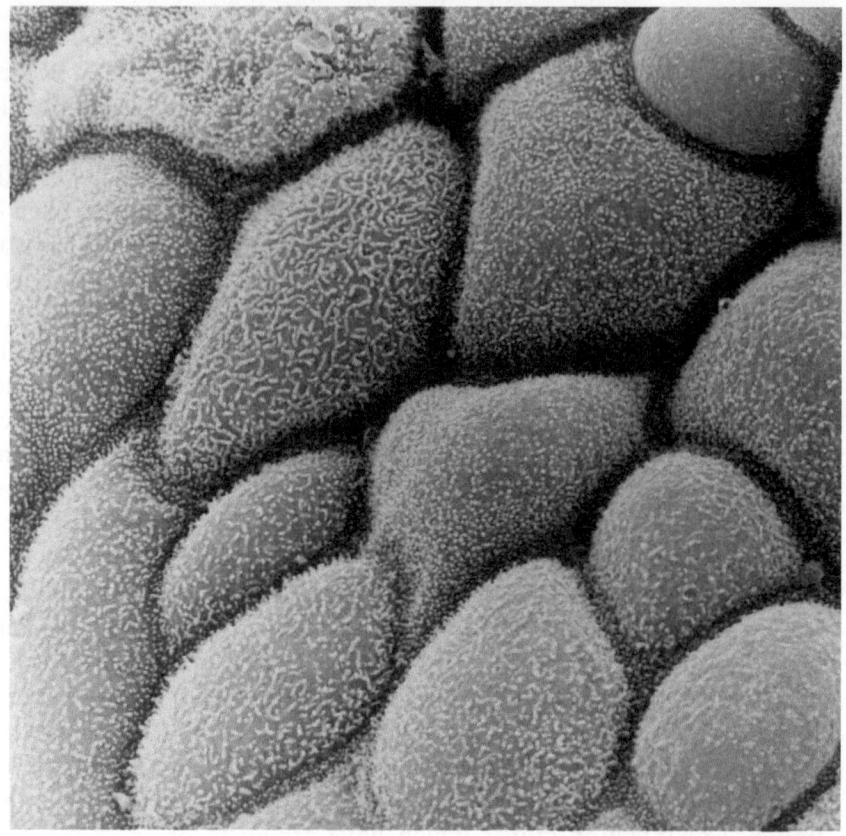

FIGURE 1.2 (a) Normal 'cobblestone' appearance of transitional bladder epithelium SEM × 2000.

penetrate into the deep layers of the bladder wall, causing chronic inflammatory change[14]. Patients in whom this occurs are characteristically:

1. Elderly women with a history of a lifetime of cystitis, often extending back into the preantibiotic era.

2. Patients of either sex who have been catheterized for any length of time.

3. Patients with the inevitable bacteriuria of neuropathic bladder, ileal bladder or other urostomies, or vesico-colic fistula.

14

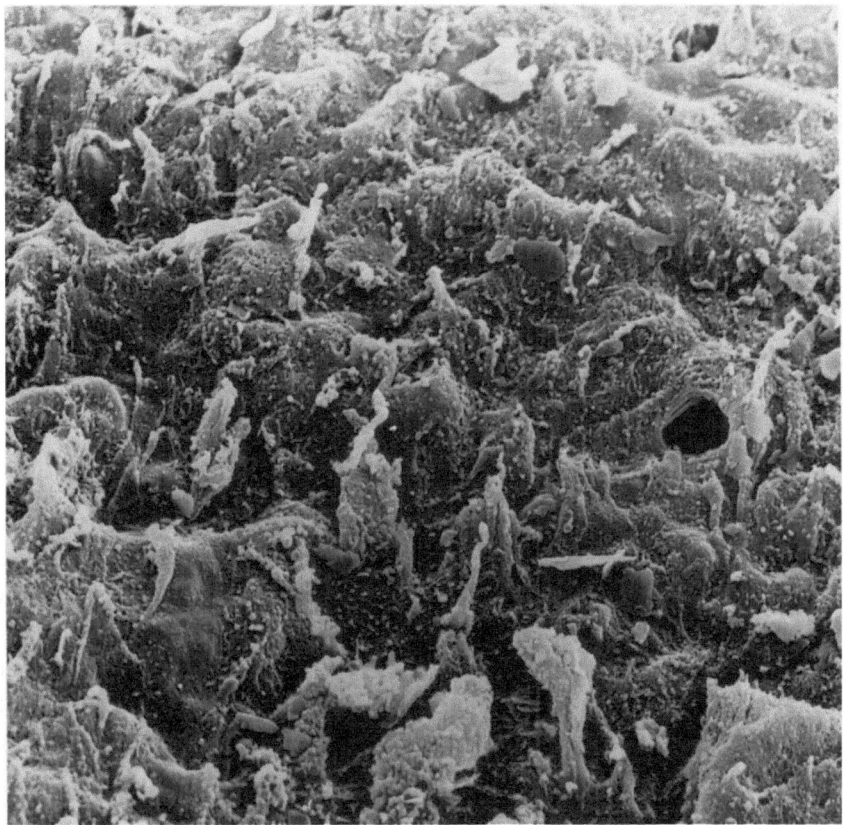

FIGURE 1.2 (b) Grossly disrupted bladder epithelium from a patient with chronic cystitis. (Photographs by S. T. Moss and P. J. Pead)

4. Patients, usually women, in whom bladder infection with fastidious organisms has developed. This condition, in the past, has remained undetected and has become chronic and deep seated. The term 'interstitial cystitis' has been applied to it. There is some recent evidence[15] that it may, in fact, result from extension of infection with such organisms from the proximal urethra and trigone, and may represent the later stages of urethral syndrome.

Prostatitis and epididymo-orchitis

There is evidence that infection of the male lower urinary tract and adjacent structures is commoner than is generally believed[16]. Such infection, although it may involve the bladder, does not always do so, and may be confined to the urethra and prostate, occasionally with retrograde spread to the epididymis and testis. Chronic inflammatory change will occur in any of these structures if:

1. There is a predisposing cause, such as an indwelling catheter or urethral stricture.

2. The antibacterial agent given for the acute infection does not effectively penetrate prostatic tissue. This will be considered later.

3. The causative organism is not detected and appropriately treated.

Since the advent of effective antigonococcal treatment this organism has become an increasingly rare cause of chronic infection; *Chlamydia trachomatis*, however, is believed to account for a proportion of the cases of prostatitis and epididymo-orchitis in younger men, and there is a growing body of evidence that *Gardnerella vaginalis* can cause such infections. Accurate bacteriological diagnosis and appropriate treatment are essential if chronic inflammation and symptoms are to be avoided.

Urethral syndrome

The aetiology of this syndrome was discussed earlier. There is some evidence that the symptoms are self-limiting in many patients, particularly if antibacterial agents, which are a major aetiological factor, are withheld[17]. Others, in particular those who are repeatedly treated with antibacterial agents, often with prolonged courses in high dosage because the symptoms fail to respond, develop chronic inflammatory changes in the paraurethral tissues. Bacteriological diagnosis and effective management undertaken in the early stages of this condition are now possible; they offer the best chance of preventing symptoms which, in the past, have troubled some women for twenty years or more.

16

Urinary tract calculi

Although 90% of urinary tract calculi have a metabolic cause, the remaining 10% are formed as the direct consequence of UTI[18], most commonly with organisms which metabolize urea in the urine, resulting in the deposition of carbonate–apatite and struvite in a friable matrix – the so-called mixed phosphatic stones. Living organisms survive in the substance of the stones, which calcify and steadily increase in size. If this occurs in the kidney, they grow to fill the renal pelvis (staghorn calculi); if in the bladder, they may eventually lodge in and obstruct the outlet. Less is known about the natural history of infection stones in the prostate, but they are commonly seen on X-rays of patients with a long history of prostatitis symptoms. Such stones were also recorded in the paraurethral tissues of women by Virchow as long ago as 1853[19]. The organisms that are characteristically associated with infection stone formation are *Proteus* spp, staphylococci (both *S. epidermidis* and *S. saprophyticus*) and *Ureaplasma urealyticum*[20].

The presence of such stones in any of the tissues of the urinary tract results in secondary inflammatory changes; in the kidney, the combination of infection and obstruction of urine drainage may lead to pyonephrosis and even psoas abscess, with septicaemia which may be fatal. Infection stones, in fact, are the only type of urinary tract calculi which are life threatening, either as a result of septicaemia or by complete destruction of the renal tissue leading to renal failure. The likelihood of the latter is increased in patients who have had repeated operations for the removal of such calculi, even nephrectomy in some cases. Early diagnosis of renal infection stones, and effective operative and antibacterial management, are therefore essential.

Use of laboratory diagnosis in the management of symptoms and identification of patients at risk from chronic inflammatory changes

There are some principles of laboratory diagnosis which, if used thoughtfully, will enable the clinician to manage the symptoms of patients with bacteriuria and to identify those who are at risk from the chronic inflammatory changes described above.

17

Children

A carefully collected and transported specimen of urine should be obtained from any child suspected of having UTI – those with micturition symptoms, enuresis, fever of uncertain origin, or failure to thrive. A follow-up specimen to confirm the efficacy of treatment should always be submitted. All children with persistent or recurrent infection should be subjected to urinary tract investigation, and many experts in the field consider that investigation is indicated after a single infection. The nature and extent of such investigations is controversial at present, and it may be some years before careful studies of the newer imaging techniques now available provide an answer to the question. A finding of apparently 'sterile' pyuria in a child who was not on antibacterial treatment at the time of specimen collection should not be ignored. Infection with fastidious organisms in childhood is rare; it usually indicates an underlying pathological condition in which such organisms have been enabled to survive in the relatively low oxygen tension of chronically inflamed tissue. A further specimen with a request for culture for fastidious organisms should be submitted, and urinary tract investigation undertaken.

Adult women

Clearly, UTI is so common in adult women that urine culture for every episode, and urinary tract investigation of all such patients, would be unnecessary and impracticable.

There is good evidence that the majority of recurrences of UTI are reinfections rather than relapses; in reinfection, the previous infection has resolved and the patient has succumbed to a further infection, whereas, with relapse or persistence of infection, the initial infection has not resolved. Reinfections characteristically occur at intervals of 3 months or more, whereas relapses manifest themselves immediately or soon after cessation of treatment, and persistent infection remains despite treatment. The patient with relapsing or persistent infection is likely to have an underlying cause for, or focus of, infection, and requires investigation; the patient with recurrences due to reinfection is unlikely to have such a condition, and requires investigation and specialist management only if the symptoms recur so frequently that they become a nuisance. Therefore:

1. A single episode of symptoms, or isolated episodes occurring rarely, may be treated without MSU culture.

2. Repeated episodes of symptoms should not be treated without MSU culture, although, if the symptoms are severe, empirical treatment may be started after the specimen has been collected. Modern methods of MSU culture can distinguish between symptoms due to bacterial cystitis (usually with aerobic organisms, but rarely with fastidious bacteria which may only be detected by additional culture methods) and those due to urethral syndrome. Management of these syndromes is quite different and will be discussed below. Problems arise particularly with those patients who suffer from both conditions; MSU culture, and withholding of antibacterial treatment until the result is available, is mandatory in such patients.

3. In patients with inevitable bacteriuria – those with long-term indwelling catheters, neuropathic bladders, urostomies – urine culture should be undertaken only when they develop a clinical indication for treatment, for example if they become feverish, generally unwell or confused. Provided the urine is cultured only at such times and antibacterial treatment is not given when they are well, the bacterial flora will remain sensitive, and episodes of clinical infection requiring treatment can be easily and effectively managed. There is no advantage in monitoring the bacteriological state of the urine of such patients at regular intervals; the flora is usually mixed, it may include several bacterial species and its make-up is constantly changing. The current bacteria and their sensitivities to antibacterial agents can only be determined by urine culture at the time of the episode of clinical illness. Much unnecessary work is expected of laboratories in this field. Efforts to restrict it to the appropriate occasions are of benefit to the laboratory and to the patients, who are spared much unnecessary, and sometimes dangerous, antibacterial treatment.

Adult men

1. MSU microscopy and culture should be undertaken in all men who present with symptoms suggestive of urinary or prostatic infection, and the efficacy of treatment should be checked by a follow-up specimen.

2. If apparently 'sterile' pyuria is found in a specimen from a male patient not on treatment, or if the symptoms persist after anti-bacterial treatment, a further MSU should be cultured by methods capable of detecting fastidious organisms.

3. If both aerobic and fastidious organism culture are negative, and pyuria or symptoms persist, the possibility of chlamydial infection may be assumed (at present, laboratory detection of chlamydial infection is not widely available except in genitourinary medicine clinics) and appropriate treatment, usually a tetracycline, given for 10 days.

4. If an MSU taken after empirical tetracycline still shows pyuria, but yields negative cultures for aerobes and fastidious pathogens, the possibility of tuberculous infection should be considered. Three early morning urine specimens should be cultured for *Mycobacterium* spp.

5. Urethral catheterization for surgery, in particular for prosta-tectomy, predisposes to infection of the bladder, urethra and pros-tatic residue. Antibacterial agents are often given perioperatively, and selection of resistant organisms in the urethral flora may result. Increasingly, male patients are subject postoperatively to troublesome infections with fastidious species, such as coryne-bacteria, and these may be multiresistant. They must be detected by appropriate culture methods after catheter removal, or if the patient becomes clinically unwell while catheterized; appropriate antibacterial treatment given for the length of time required to eradicate tissue infection is necessary. This will be considered below.

Selection of patients for urinary tract investigation

It follows from much of what has been written above that there are certain clinical and bacteriological pointers which can help the clinician to select those patients who may be at risk from the serious consequences of UTI, or who might benefit from specialist management.

TABLE 1.1   Some important indications for investigation of children with UTI or pyuria

---

Recurrent or persistent UTI
Proteus infection in girls
UTI with fever or failure to thrive
UTI with enuresis
UTI with an unusual organism, e.g. *Staphylococcus aureus,*
  S. epidermidis, Pseudomonas sp.
UTI with a resistant organism
UTI with hypertension
Apparently 'sterile' pyuria or UTI with a fastidious organism

---

Table 1.1 lists some important factors which should prompt hospital referral and investigation of children with UTI or pyuria; Table 1.2 does the same for adults. Of course, not all the patients who require investigation will be identified by the use of these criteria, and many others, in particular adult women with frequent and troublesome episodes of urinary symptoms, can benefit from specialist investigation and management.

TABLE 1.2   Some important indications for investigation of adults with UTI or pyuria

---

Persistent or relapsing UTI
Haematuria persisting after successful treatment of UTI
UTI with hypertension (except in the elderly)
UTI with resistant or unusual organisms (except in elderly or catheterized
  patients)
Recurrent or persistent *Proteus* infection
An attack of acute pyelonephritis, or UTI with fever

ANTIBACTERIAL AGENTS AND MANAGEMENT PROTOCOLS

The well-tried and inexpensive oral agents – nitrofurantoin, co-trimoxazole and amoxycillin – still provide the mainstay of treatment. In areas where laboratory practice and communications with clinicians have been good, the great majority of aerobic urinary pathogens have remained sensitive to at least two of these agents[21,22]. However, in recent years, the widespread use of ampicillin/amoxycillin in the community has resulted in a marked reduction in the percentage of urinary pathogens sensitive to these agents[21]. The use of trimethoprin alone – rather than in combination with sulphamethoxazole in co-trimoxazole – has coincided with a dramatic rise in the level of resistance to this agent. As a consequence, some of the cephalosporins, Augmentin (a combination of amoxycillin and clavulanic acid) and the new quinolones (ciprofloxacin, norfloxacin) are being used increasingly for oral treatment of UTI. Parenteral treatment is seldom required; the agents used are those in general use for treatment of Gram-negative or Gram-positive organisms, as appropriate. Detailed discussion of the antibacterial spectrum and appropriate use of all these agents would be out of place here, but they have been summarized elsewhere[23].

Antibacterial treatment protocols

There are clearly-defined and specific protocols for the management or prevention of UTI, each having its particular uses, but misunderstandings are widespread in this field, and it is worthwhile considering these protocols in some detail.

All patients with UTI, whatever treatment regimen is used, should be instructed in the importance of the washout mechanism in prevention of infection. They should be encouraged to drink well and to empty their bladder, using double micturition, at least every 2 hours and after sexual intercourse, if appropriate.

Single dose or short course therapy

Oral antibacterial agents may be used in single therapeutic dosage or for 2–3 days. There is no evidence that use in higher-than-normal therapeutic dosage is any more effective. This regimen is useful for treatment of attacks of acute cystitis in adult women. Bacteriological follow up is essential in order to detect treatment failure. It is particularly useful in the management of proven aerobic infection in women who are also subject to attacks of urethral syndrome, and are therefore at greater risk from selection of lactobacilli in the urethra by prolonged antibacterial treatment. Single-dose or short-course treatment should never be used for children, adult males or patients with acute pyelonephritis or fever, in whom tissue infection is likely and may have serious consequences.

Standard 5-day therapy

Five days' treatment with an oral agent in therapeutic dosage is the mainstay of the management of UTI in children and adult women. Longer courses in therapeutic dosage have no advantage over 5 days; they have the considerable disadvantage of increasing the likelihood of side effects and selection of a resistant flora in the bowel, vagina and urethra.

Treatment of adult males

UTI in adult males either originates in the prostate, with extension to the bladder, or is confined to the prostate. Treatment, therefore, must assume tissue infection, and an agent which penetrates prostatic tissue effectively must be used. For Gram-negative infections, either co-trimoxazole, a tetracycline such as doxycycline, or a quinolone such as ciprofloxacin, should be given, according to the sensitivity of the organism. Erythromycin is a useful additional alternative for treatment of Gram-positive infections. The minimum duration of treatment should be 10 days; a 14-day course is sometimes necessary. Frequent

23

recurrences or relapses may require a low-dose prophylactic or suppressive regimen (see below).

Low-dose prophylaxis or suppression

The indications for low-dose prophylactic or suppressive regimens are shown in Table 1.3. In the majority of patients the purpose of such regimens is to prevent further recurrences of infection, preventing

TABLE 1.3   Indications for long-term low-dose prophylactic or suppressive antibacterial regimens

---

Children
  Recurrent UTI
  V–u reflux with or without renal scarring

Adults
  Frequent recurrent symptomatic infections
  Persistent or relapsing infections in patients with stones, renal scarring
    or prostatitis
  Pregnancy in women with UTI or a history of childhood UTI or recurrent
    infection

---

tissue damage and allowing recovery of normal defence mechanisms. In a minority of patients, eradication of infection is impossible, for example in some patients with infection stones or some men with persistent infection in scarred prostatic tissue; suppression of infection in the urine itself by a long-term low-dose regimen can prevent stone growth[24] or extension of tissue damage.

The prophylactic regimen should be preceded, if infection is present, by a 5-day therapeutic course of an appropriate agent followed immediately by prophylaxis. The antibacterial agents suitable for use in prophylaxis are those with a wide spectrum which are well absorbed, excreted in the urine and not particularly liable to select resistance in the commensal flora of the bowel, vagina or urethra. For these reasons, the two agents that have proved valuable and effective over the course of time are nitrofurantoin and co-trimoxazole. The principal limitation of the former is the fact that it is ineffective against *Proteus* spp. and therefore inappropriate for use in young boys (in whom *Proteus* is the

24

commonest urinary pathogen[13]) or in patients with infection stones. In recent years, resistance has developed to co-trimoxazole, particularly when trimethoprim alone has been used[25]. Two of the oral cephalosporins, cephradine[26] and cefaclor[27], have been reported as useful for this purpose; again the limitation of the former agent is that most isolates of *Proteus* are resistant to it. Neither agent, of course, penetrates prostatic tissue and use in adult males would therefore be unsuitable.

The prophylactic dosage of all these agents is one quarter of the treatment dose appropriate to the age and sex of the patient. It is given once daily, last thing at night in order to ensure a concentration in the bladder urine overnight when the washout mechanism is inactive. The published evidence indicates that prophylactic regimens should be continued at least until the patient has been free of infection for one year; shorter periods of prophylaxis are often followed by recurrence of infection. Urine culture should be undertaken at regular intervals – at least 3-monthly – and appropriate treatment given if infection recurs. More than one recurrence of infection while on a prophylactic regimen is a reason for reconsidering the use of prophylaxis, and to abandon it if it seems likely to be unsuccessful. Successful prophylaxis may need to be continued for longer than one year, sometimes indefinitely, in some patients – for example those with infection stones, extensive renal scarring or very recalcitrant prostatitis. Low-dose prophylaxis should never be attempted in patients with inevitable bacteriuria – those with long-term indwelling catheters, neuropathic bladders or urostomies; the only effect of attempts at such management is to select a resistant flora in the urine, rendering treatment of episodes of clinical infection difficult and sometimes impossible.

Short-term prophylaxis

This is the use of antibacterial agents in therapeutic dosage over a short period of time to prevent infection which might occur as a result of instrumentation or an operative procedure. Definite indications for such prophylaxis are:

1. Catheterization for investigations such as micturating cysto-urethrography or urodynamic studies.

2. Dilatation of, or operation on, a urethral stricture.

There is also evidence that short-term prophylaxis may be effective in preventing UTI in patients undergoing urological or gynaecological surgery necessitating catheterization. Provided that the period of catheterization does not exceed 3–5 days, the prophylaxis may be effective; if catheterization is prolonged, infection will inevitably occur, and the bacteria will be resistant if antibacterial prophylaxis has been given. A complicating factor in determining the advisability of attempts at prophylaxis in patients undergoing surgery is the necessity for treatment of other perioperative complications, such as chest infection.

Therapeutic dosage is required for short-term prophylaxis; regimens vary from a single intravenous injection to oral dosage continued for a few days. The agents used, either singly or in combination, must be chosen in the light of existing infection, if present, and the spectrum of potential pathogens.

Management protocols for some special groups of patients

The various regimens described above should be chosen as appropriate to the clinical circumstances of the individual patient. In addition, there are some other aspects of management of UTI in particular groups of patients which have been worked out or improved in recent years.

Patients with infection stones

The management of such patients requires close co-operation between laboratory, surgeon and physician. A carefully monitored co-ordination of surgery and antibacterial treatment offers the best outlook to patients with this serious, and potentially lethal, condition. Early diagnosis, often because the clinician is alerted to the possibility by persistent or repeated UTI with urea-splitting organisms, such as *Proteus* spp. or staphylococci, enables surgery to be undertaken at a stage before the renal damage due to obstruction has occurred (Figure 1.3). It is interesting that many patients with infection stones, even of large staghorn dimensions, are completely free from urinary symptoms. With modern developments in urological practice, it is now possible to fragment some renal stones by extracorporeal shock-wave lithotripsy, and to remove others by the percutaneous route. Open operations for stone removal, and partial or total nephrectomy for stones are now only rarely necessary. All surgical procedures for removal or fragmentation of infection stones must be covered by appropriate antibacterial therapy. The risk of spread of living organisms from the substance of the stone into the renal tissues and the bloodstream is high, and can be life threatening. Furthermore, after surgical removal, the natural history of stone formation of this type must be remembered; it is very unlikely that every fragment of friable stone material and every organism has been removed surgically, and the risk of further stone formation is high. Effective perioperative antibacterial cover must be followed by low-dose prophylaxis, with careful bacteriological supervision, until the urine has remained sterile for one year and there has been no further stone formation.

Late diagnosis, very large stones, or recurrent stones in kidneys already subjected to extensive surgery may render some or all of the surgical options for removal impossible. In these circumstances, every effort must be made to keep the urine sterile by low-dose antibacterial suppression (see above), thus preventing stone growth and spread of infection. However, should it prove impossible to keep the urine sterile in this way, the prophylactic agent should be stopped; antibacterial treatment should then be reserved for episodes of clinical infection. Both the patient and their general practitioner should be alerted to the need for prompt treatment, and hospital admission if the patient has evidence of septicaemia.

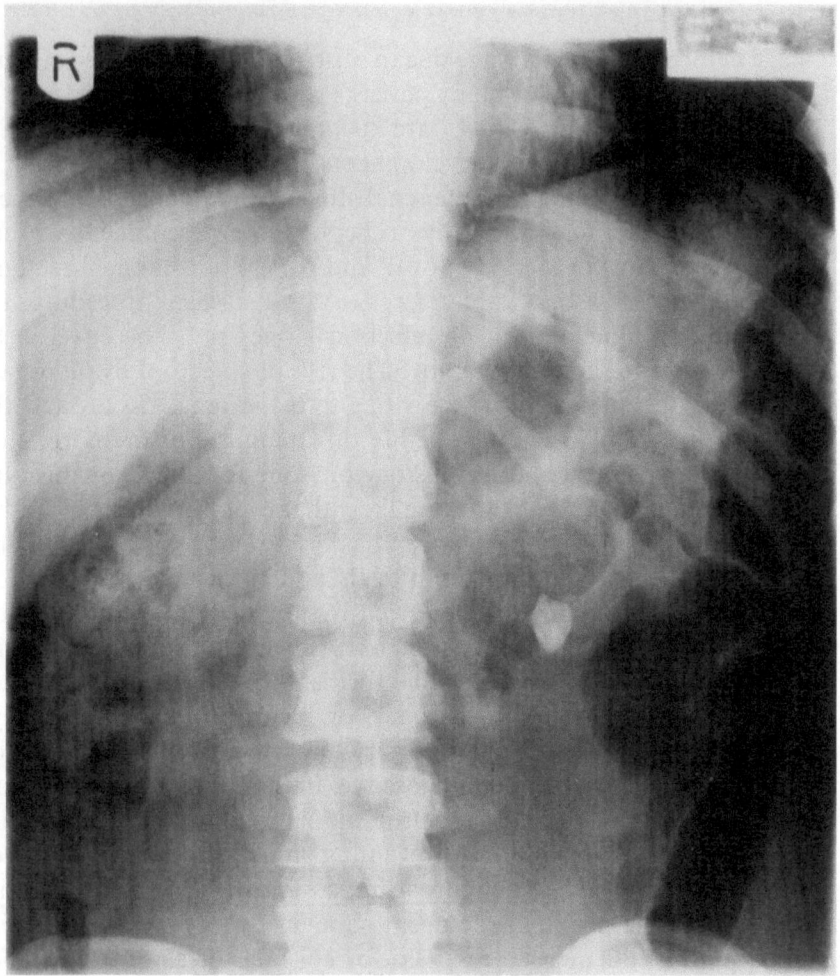

FIGURE 1.3   (a) Plain abdominal X-ray of patient with infection stones;
large stone in lower pole of left kidney, small stone in lower pole of right
kidney

Inevitable bacteriuria

It has already been mentioned that bacteriuria is inevitable in some
clinical situations. The principal determining factors are either that
the washout mechanism, which is the major physiological protection
against infection, is impaired, or that there is an easy direct route by

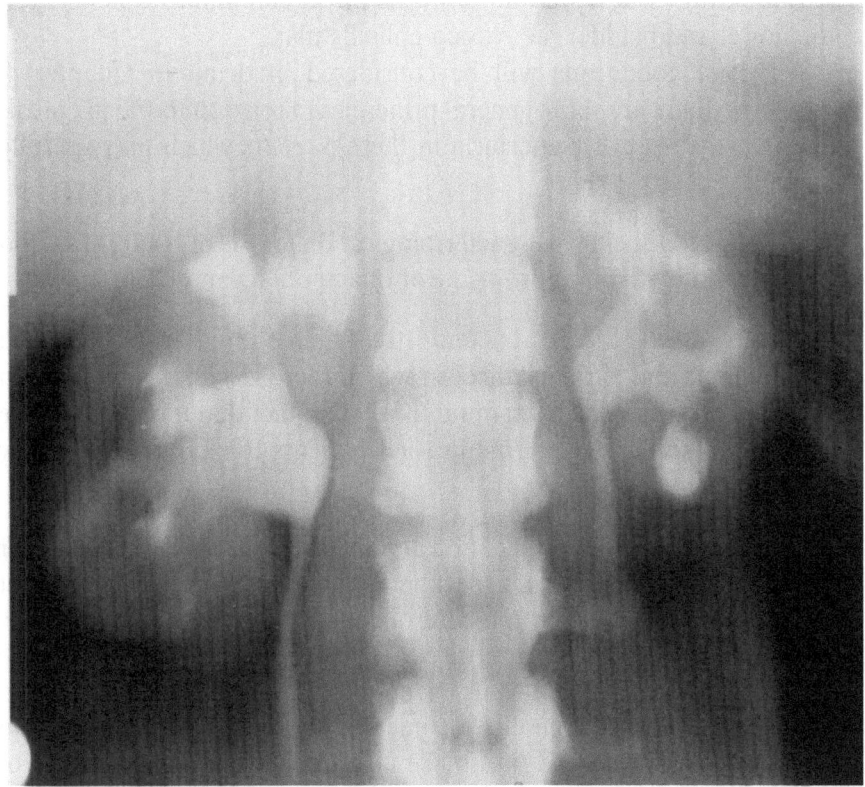

FIGURE 1.3 (b) IVU with tomography at 10 minutes of the same patient showing the changes of bilateral chronic pyelonephritis. The left kidney is small and there is bilateral loss of renal cortex and clubbing of the calyces

which organisms can gain access to the bladder. The first group comprises those patients with neurological impairment of bladder function due to diseases of the nervous system, such as multiple sclerosis, to the neurological complications of general diseases, such as diabetes, or to congenital, traumatic, or neoplastic damage to the spinal cord, and those with ileal bladders. The second group consists of those patients with indwelling catheters (the weight of evidence is that the infecting bacteria ascend along the moist outer surface of the catheter and colonize not only the bladder but also the prostate and paraurethral tissues), and those with a direct communication between the bowel and bladder, i.e. vesico-colic fistula.

All these conditions will be considered in detail in Chapter 4. However, there are some general principles in relation to the diagnosis and management of bacteriuria in these patients which may usefully be set out here:

1. The usual principles of bacteriological diagnosis of bacteriuria and treatment with an appropriate antibacterial agent do not apply.

2. Urine culture and antibacterial treatment should be restricted to occasions and circumstances in which there is a clinical indication for treatment, bearing in mind the certain fact that it is not possible to maintain a sterile urine in such patients for longer than a few days.

3. If there is a clinical indication for treatment, e.g. fever, rigors, or acute confusion, a urine specimen should be collected by the best method available – in the case of a patient with an ileal bladder, the stoma should be carefully catheterized. Urine from drainage bags should never be sent for culture. The request form should make it clear that there is a clinical indication for treatment, and the laboratory should set up primary sensitivity tests of a range of agents suitable to cover the likely bacterial flora, which is almost certain to be mixed. Empirical antibacterial treatment should be started, and altered if necessary, in the light of the sensitivity report.

4. Antibacterial treatment should never be given to such patients when they are well, or for longer than is needed to obtain clinical cure of an episode of systemic infection. The only consequence of prolonged treatment is the selection of resistant organisms and a mixed flora, making treatment, when necessary, more difficult.

5. The major risk to these patients is ascending sepsis in the urinary tract, either pyelonephritic scarring or the development of infection stones in the kidneys or bladder. The likelihood of scarring may be reduced by reserving antibacterial treatment for episodes of clinical illness, which can then be treated promptly and effectively

because the organisms are likely to be sensitive. Infection stones are amenable to surgical treatment if they are detected at an early stage, and removal will help to preserve renal tissue and function. An annual plain film of the abdomen, therefore, is advisable in patients with inevitable bacteriuria.

6. Attempts at low-dose prophylaxis are always unsuccessful and harmful for the reasons given above. Such management is contra-indicated.

All the above principles apply equally to patients who undertake intermittent self-catheterization, a very useful modern advance in the management of some patients with neuropathic bladders or incontinence. It must be accepted that the bladder urine will be infected for most of the time; experience has shown, however, that the regular drainage of the bladder obtained by this procedure lessens the likelihood of ascending infection and septicaemia. Antibacterial treatment should be reserved for episodes of clinical infection.

Urinary tract infection in patients with renal failure

UTI occurs in such patients for one of two reasons:

1. In about 20% of the patients coming on to dialysis programmes, the primary cause of renal failure is an infection-related disease, usually chronic pyelonephritic scarring secondary to v–u reflux, or infection stones.

2. Secondary bacteriuria may develop in patients with advanced renal failure who have a low urinary output and empty their bladders infrequently. This is due to stasis and impairment of the washout mechanism.

In the first group – those with infection-related primary disease – it is possible to preserve renal function by appropriate antibacterial treatment and prophylaxis, provided the degree of renal failure is only mild or moderate. Once the serum creatinine level has reached about $400 \, \mu\text{mol L}^{-1}$, there is little evidence that control of infection is effective in preserving function; in these patients, antibacterial treatment

31

should be reserved for the episodes of clinical infection that such patients are likely to develop during the course of dialysis and transplantation, to which they will progress.

In the second group, the difficulty of diagnosing UTI is considerable. Patients who pass only small volumes of urine occasionally are unable to provide a good MSU, and the need for accurate diagnosis may warrant collection of a catheter specimen. The urine of such patients should not be cultured unless they have clinical evidence of UTI; it will usually yield a mixed bacterial growth, and antibacterial treatment will only be harmful.

COVERT BACTERIURIA

This term has been used interchangeably with 'asymptomatic bacteriuria'; it has been applied to bacteriuria detected in patients at times when they are free of symptoms related to micturition. There has been much controversy over the years as to its significance, how it should be regarded by the clinician, and whether either antibacterial treatment or urinary tract investigation is indicated. If these questions are to be answered, it is first necessary to consider the possible explanations for the finding.

1. Some bacteria may be of an insufficiently virulent type to adhere to or invade tissue, and, therefore, they may not give rise to symptoms.

2. Covert bacteriuria might be a phase in the natural history of patients with recurrent or persistent cystitis. Micturition symptoms are thought to be due to acute inflammatory changes in the bladder, urethra or paraurethral tissues. It is well known that the symptoms of an acute attack of cystitis will disappear after a few days, even if the bacteriuria is untreated and persists.

3. Covert bacteriuria might be due to the presence of bacteria elsewhere in the urinary tract, other than the bladder, for example in renal scars or infection stones. Such infection may not be accompanied by acute inflammatory changes in the bladder and, therefore, may not give rise to micturition symptoms.

32

4. Covert bacteriuria may be only apparently asymptomatic. Many patients, especially elderly women who have experienced a lifetime of cystitis, often going back to the preantibiotic era, have come to accept some frequency, nocturia and even incontinence as normal.

5. Many patients with the inevitable bacteriuria which occurs with long-term indwelling catheters, ileal bladders, neuropathic bladders and intermittent self-catheterization, are apparently free from urinary symptoms for most of the time.

6. Bacteriuria and infection-related diseases of the urinary tract are not uncommon amongst the physically and mentally handicapped. They may be unable to complain of symptoms.

Bacteriuria with non-virulent organisms

It is recognized that the establishment of bacteria in the urinary tract is regulated by a variety of bacterial virulence factors and is determined by the balance between such factors and host defences. The evidence for the many factors involved in this interaction was recently reviewed by Winberg[28]. One determinant of virulence, possession of P-fimbriae by certain strains of *Escherichia coli*, has been shown to be important in some clinical situations, for example the first attack of acute pyelonephritis in children[29]. However, although much lower percentages of P-fimbriated strains were isolated from children with asymptomatic bacteriuria, non-fimbriated strains were also isolated from children with recurrent or chronic pyelonephritis. It has been suggested that treatment of bacteriuria with apparently non-virulent strains may open the way to recurrence of infection with more virulent ones; this is sometimes used as an argument against treatment of covert bacteriuria in children. However, the conflicting evidence in this field suggests that, at present, this is an unwise assumption. Furthermore, tests for detecting virulence factors are not yet in general use.

Covert bacteriuria as a phase in the natural history of recurrent UTI and the possibility of persistent infection in the urinary tract or adjacent tissues

The evidence that this may occur, both in children and adults, is undisputed. Children and adult women identified as bacteriuric in screening programmes at times when they are apparently symptom free may give a history of episodes of micturition-related symptoms; others subsequently develop symptomatic infections[30]. It is wise, therefore, to assume that covert bacteriuria, whether detected in screening programmes or on admission to hospital for other reasons, is a significant finding. It is an indication of previous or longstanding infection and the reason for this should be sought. In an interesting small study of bacteriuric women in general practice some years ago[31], Manners and his colleagues showed that radiological abnormalities were detected on IVU in 48% of the patients with covert bacteriuria, but only in 4% of those with recurrent symptomatic bacterial cystitis. It is certainly the experience of clinicians who look after patients, both adults and children, with chronic pyelonephritic scarring or infection stones that many such patients are completely free from micturition symptoms. Even if radiological investigations reveal no abnormality, an attempt should be made to eradicate the bacteriuria by appropriate treatment followed by low-dose prophylaxis if it recurs. Persistent bacteriuria in women or children with normal radiology suggests the possibility of deep-seated bladder wall infection. The lengths to which diagnosis and attempts at treatment should be taken must be determined by the age of the patient. Children, and young women for whom sexual activity is in the future, are at risk from ascending infection if the bacteriuria is allowed to persist. In middle life, there is the additional risk of scarring and contraction of the bladder, which gives rise to severe and unpleasant symptoms. Covert bacteriuria is rare in young boys and adult males who have not been catheterized or instrumented. It invariably indicates underlying pathology which should be sought and treated.

Covert bacteriuria in the elderly

This is common in both sexes, in women who have suffered cystitis for many years and in men who have been instrumented for operative procedures, most commonly prostatectomy. Bacteriuria in these patients is often due to well-established tissue infection, and it is not easily eradicated by antibacterial therapy. The need for urinary tract investigation and for attempts at treatment must be determined by the age and general condition of the patient.

Symptom-free patients with inevitable bacteriuria

The management of such patients has already been discussed. Severe symptoms or systemic upset are the only indications for antibacterial treatment. One radiological investigation that can be usefully performed in all but the very elderly is an annual plain abdominal X-ray to detect infection stone formation.

Bacteriuria screening programmes

Informed opinion does not, at present, favour screening programmes for detection of bacteriuria in children. If significant urinary tract abnormalities are to be detected and progressive disease prevented, such screening must start in early childhood, when not all children attend places, such as nursery schools, where screening could be carried out. Effective action on the results of screening necessitates a greater degree of understanding and co-operation between the organizers of the screening programme, the general practitioners and paediatricians than is often available. There is an annual incidence of bacteriuria of about 1% in girls, bacteriuria may be intermittent, and v–u reflux may persist into adolescence. Screening, therefore, must be repeated at regular intervals and it is an expensive procedure. Children at risk from bacteriuria are better identified by awareness on the part of general practitioners, and easy availability of reliable MSU culture for children who present to them with symptoms or systemic upset.

The weight of evidence available at present suggests that screening of women for bacteriuria in early pregnancy is justified. Up to 5% of pregnant women are found to be bacteriuric in the first trimester; treatment will cure the majority of these infections and considerably lower the incidence of acute pyelonephritis in the second trimester.

Screening in pregnancy also provides an opportunity for identification, by careful history taking, of those women in whom infection dates back to childhood or is difficult to eradicate. These women should be subjected to urinary tract investigation after the puerperium. All these advantages of pregnancy bacteriuria screening are lost, however, if communications between patient, general practitioner and obstetrician are poor; programmes in which audit shows that the benefits are lost through poor communications should be discontinued.

REFERENCES

1. Kass, E. H. (1956). Asymptomatic infections of the urinary tract. *Trans. Assoc. Am. Physicians*, **69**, 56–63
2. Kass, E. H. (1957). Bacteriuria and the diagnosis of infections of the urinary tract. *Arch. Intern. Med.*, **100**, 709–714
3. Kincaid-Smith, P. and Fairley, K. F. (1965). Diagnosis of urinary tract infection. *Hosp. Med.*, **1**, 993–998
4. Gallagher, D. J. A., Montgomerie, J. Z. and North, J. D. K. (1965). Acute infections of the urinary tract and the urethral syndrome in general practice. *Br. Med. J.*, **1**, 622–626
5. Stamm, W. E., Wagner, K. F., Amsel, R., Alexander, E. R., Turck, W., Counts, K. K. and Holmes, G. W. (1980). Causes of the acute urethral syndrome in women. *N. Engl. J. Med.*, **303**, 409–415
6. Maskell, R. and Polak, A. (1973). Bacteriological facilities for the diagnosis of urinary infection in general practice. In Brumfitt, W. and Asscher, A. W. (eds.) *Urinary Tract Infection*, pp. 3–10. (London: Oxford University Press)
7. Maskell, R. (1986). Are fastidious organisms an important cause of dysuria and frequency? – the case for. In Asscher, A. W. and Brumfitt, W. (eds.) *Microbial Diseases in Nephrology*, pp. 1–18 (Chichester: John Wiley and Sons)
8. Papapetropoulou, M. and Pappas, A. (1987). The acute urethral syndrome in routine practice. *J. Infect.*, **14**, 113–118
9. Barr, J. G., Ritchie, J. W. K., Henry, O., El Sheik, M. and El Deeb, K. (1985). Microaerophilic/anaerobic bacteria as a cause of urinary tract infection in pregnancy. *Br. J. Obstet. Gynaecol.*, **92**, 506–510
10. Wu, T. C., Williams, E. C., Koo, S. Y. and Mac Lowry, J. D. (1985). Evaluation of three bacteriuria screening methods in a clinical research hospital. *J. Clin. Microbiol.*, **21**, 796–799
11. Wilkins, E. G. L., Ratcliffe, J. G. and Roberts, C. (1985). Leucocyte esterase-nitrite screening method for pyuria and bacteriuria. *J. Clin. Pathol.*, **38**, 1342–1345
12. Maskell, R., Pead, L., Pead, P. J. and Balsdon, M. (1984). Chlamydial infection and urinary symptoms. *Br. J. Vener. Dis.*, **60**, 65
13. Maskell, R. M. and Pead, L. J. (1976). Urinary infection in children in general practice: a laboratory view. *J. Hyg. Camb.*, **77**, 291–298

14. Elliott, T. S. J., Slack, R. C. B. and Bishop, M. C. (1984). Scanning electron microscopy of human bladder mucosa in acute and chronic urinary tract infection. *Br. J. Urol.*, **56,** 38–43
15. Wilkins, E. G. L., Payne, S. R., Pead, P. J., Moss, S. T. and Maskell, R. (1988). Interstitial cystitis and urethral syndrome: a possible answer. *Br. J. Urol.* (in press)
16. Clarke, M., Pead, L. and Mashell, R. (1985). Urinary infection in adult men: a laboratory perspective. *Br. J. Urol.*, **57,** 222–226
17. Maskell, R., Pead, L. and Sanderson, R. A. (1983), Fastidious bacteria and the urethral syndrome: a 2-year clinical and bacteriological study of 51 women. *Lancet*, **2,** 1277–1280
18. Rose, G. A. and Harrison, R. (1974). The incidence, investigation and treatment of idiopathic hypercalciuria. *Br. J. Urol.*, **46,** 261–274
19. Virchow, R. (1853). Prostata-concretionen beim weib. *Arch. Pathol. Anat. Physiol.*, **5,** 403–406
20. Hedelin, H., Brorson, J. E., Grenabo, L. and Pettersson, S. (1984). *Ureaplasma urealyticum* and upper urinary tract stones. *Br. J. Urol.*, **56,** 244–249
21. Grüneberg, R. N. (1984). Antibiotic sensitivities of urinary pathogens, 1971–82. *J. Antimicrob. Chemother.*, **14,** 17–23
22. Maskell, R. (1988). *Urinary Tract Infection in Clinical and Laboratory Practice,* p. 51. (London: Edward Arnold)
23. Maskell, R. (1988). *Ibid.* pp. 43–67
24. Chinn, R. H., Maskell, R., Mead, J. A. and Polak, A. (1976). Renal stones and urinary infection: a study of antibiotic treatment. *Br. Med. J.*, **2,** 1411–1413
25. Brumfitt, W., Smith, G. W., Hamilton-Miller, J. M. T. and Gargan, R. A. (1985). A clinical comparison between Macrodantin and trimethoprim for prophylaxis in women with recurrent urinary infections. *J. Antimicrob. Chemother.*, **16,** 111–120
26. Brumfitt, W. and Hamilton-Miller, J. M. T. (1987). Recurrent urinary infections in women: clinical trial of cephradine as a prophylactic agent. *Infection*, **15,** 344–347
27. Maskell, R. (1988). *Urinary Tract Infection in Clinical and Laboratory Practice*, p. 62. (London: Edward Arnold)
28. Winberg, J. (1986). Balance between host defence and bacterial virulence in urinary tract infection. In Asscher, A. W. and Brumfitt, W. (eds.) *Microbial Diseases in Nephrology*, pp. 197–223. (Chichester: John Wiley and Sons)
29. Lomberg, H., Hellström, M., Jodal, U., Leffler, H., Lincoln, K. and Svanborg Edén, C. (1984). Virulence-associated traits in *Escherichia coli* causing first and recurrent episodes of urinary tract infection in children with or without vesicoureteral reflux. *J. Infect. Dis.*, **150,** 561–569
30. Asscher, A. W., Chick, S., Radford, N., Waters, W. E., Sussman, M., Joy, A. S., Evans, M., McLachlan, M. and Williams, J. E. (1973). Natural history of asymptomatic bacteriuria (ASB) in non-pregnant women. In Brumfitt, W. and Asscher, A. W. (eds.) *Urinary Tract Infection*, pp. 51–61. (London: Oxford University Press)
31. Manners, B. T. B., Grob, P. R., Dulake, C. and Grieve, N. W. T. (1973). The interrelationships of asymptomatic bacteriuria, acute bacterial pyelonephritis and bacterial cystitis in women. In Brumfitt, W. and Asscher, A. W. (eds.) *Urinary Tract Infection*, pp. 186–94. (London: Oxford University Press)

2

VESICO-URETERIC REFLUX: RECENT RESEARCH AND ITS EFFECT UPON CLINICAL PRACTICE

J. M. SMELLIE AND C. E. DAMAN WILLEMS

INTRODUCTION

Definition

Vesico-ureteric reflux (VUR) is defined as the backflow of urine from the bladder to the ureter through an incompetent vesico-ureteric valve. The recognition in the early 1960's of its association with childhood urinary tract infection (UTI) and the coarse renal scarring of chronic atrophic pyelonephritis (CPN) or reflux nephropathy (RN) has provoked a large and often controversial body of literature and has stimulated clinical and experimental research in this field. Most controversy has centred upon whether uncomplicated vesico-ureteric reflux matters and upon the most appropriate management of children found to have it.

Reflux may take place only intermittently or can be present continuously, both at rest and during micturition, and may vary from minimal incompetence, allowing reflux up to the pelvic brim in an undilated ureter, to gross reflux with dilatation of both ureter and renal pelvis, atonicity of the ureter and varying degrees of deformity of the calyces. The renal appearances depend both upon the bladder voiding pressure, which will be transmitted directly to the renal papillae if the vesico-ureteric junction (VUJ) is incompetent, and also upon the renal morphology, as scarring or hydronephrosis may already be present when VUR is first diagnosed. If compound renal papillae are present, intrarenal reflux (IRR) or calyco-tubular backflow of urine may also occur.

In view of these wide variations, it is difficult to generalize about the aetiology, significance, prognosis or, ultimately, management of vesico-ureteric reflux. Various methods of grading reflux based upon the radiological appearances have been introduced with these points in mind. Scott[1] suggested only two grades: reflux with and without dilatation. Smellie's four grades[2] include: minimal reflux, reflux extending up to the kidney on voiding only, or both at rest and on voiding, and reflux with dilatation of ureter and/or renal pelvis. In Rolleston's and the Birmingham three grade systems, Grade 2 includes all reflux extending to the kidney without dilatation[3,4]. Five grades of reflux, differentiating the degree of upper tract dilatation, have also been used[5,6]

However, it has been recognized that reflux appearances can vary in an individual and the apparent severity can be influenced by the technique used. This variability has complicated comparisons between different studies. In order to conduct a multicentre study and also to permit comparison of the results of different studies, the International Reflux Study Group not only defined five grades of reflux, but proposed a standardized technique for contrast cystography upon which these were based[7] (IRSC grading) (Figure 2.1).

Incidence

Sampson, in 1903[8], and Bumpus, in 1924[9], both drew attention to the finding of vesico-ureteric reflux and considered it pathological. Studies conducted in apparently normal uninfected infants and children showed a minimal incidence[10]. Jones and Headstream found reflux in one of a hundred apparently normal infants and children[11]. Lich et al. studied 28 infants within 48 hours of birth. There was no reflux in 26 but there was reflux in 2 infants with urinary infection[12].

The precise incidence of reflux remains unknown because the diagnosis of VUR still depends upon invasive techniques. It is hoped that

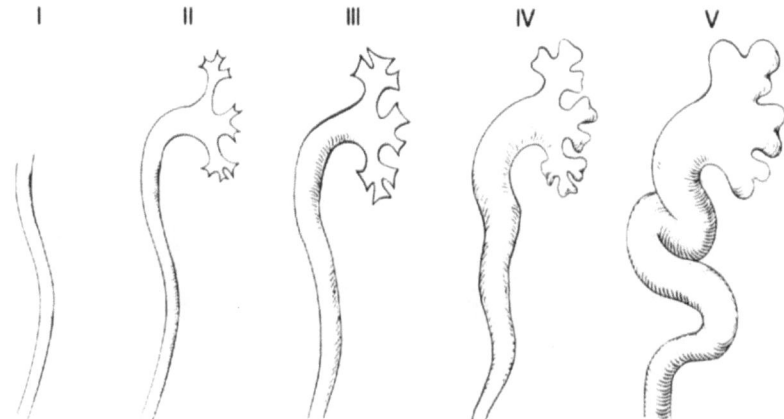

I   II   III   IV   V

FIGURE 2.1   Grades of reflux (International classification)[116]

  I. Ureter only.

 II. Ureter, pelvis and calyces; no dilatation. Normal calyceal fornices.

III. Mild or moderate dilatation and/or tortuosity of the ureter, and mild or moderate dilatation of renal pelvis but no, or only slight, blunting of the fornices.

IV. Moderate dilatation and/or tortuosity of ureter and moderate dilatation of renal pelvis and calyces; complete obliteration of sharp angle of fornices but maintenance of papillary impressions in majority of calyces.

 V. Gross dilatation and tortuosity of ureter; gross dilatation of renal pelvis and calyces; papillary impressions are no longer visible in majority of calyces

the follow up with cystography of infants considered to have urinary tract dilatation on antenatal ultrasound, and who are not subsequently shown to have urinary tract obstruction, will provide further information (Figures 2.2a and b).

VUR is usually diagnosed during investigation of children with UTI and is the commonest abnormal radiological finding in them, occurring in about one-third of patients in most series[4,13–16]. This is true both in children with symptomatic infection and in those with bacteriuria found on screening[17,18]. Allowing for the difference in frequency of urinary tract infection between the sexes, a similar proportion of males and females with UTI have VUR. Racial differences have been noted, for example Kunin *et al.* found that, in bacteriuric

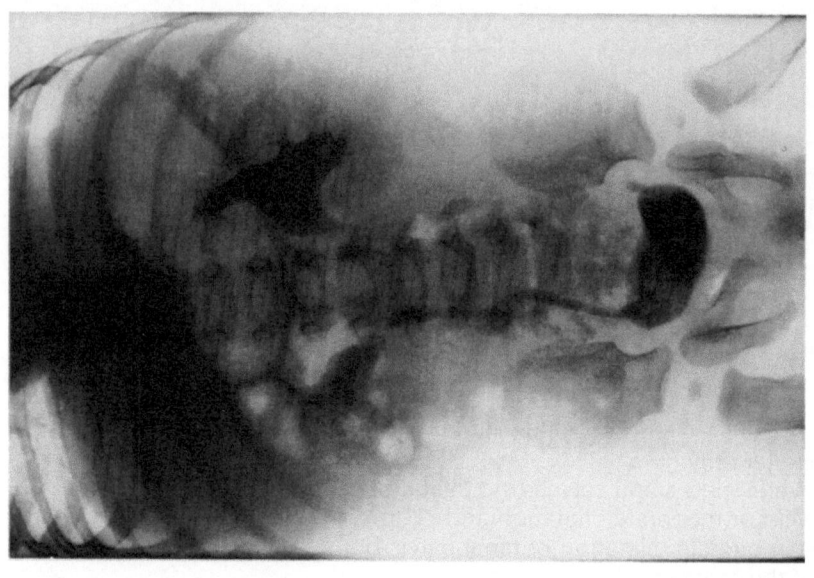

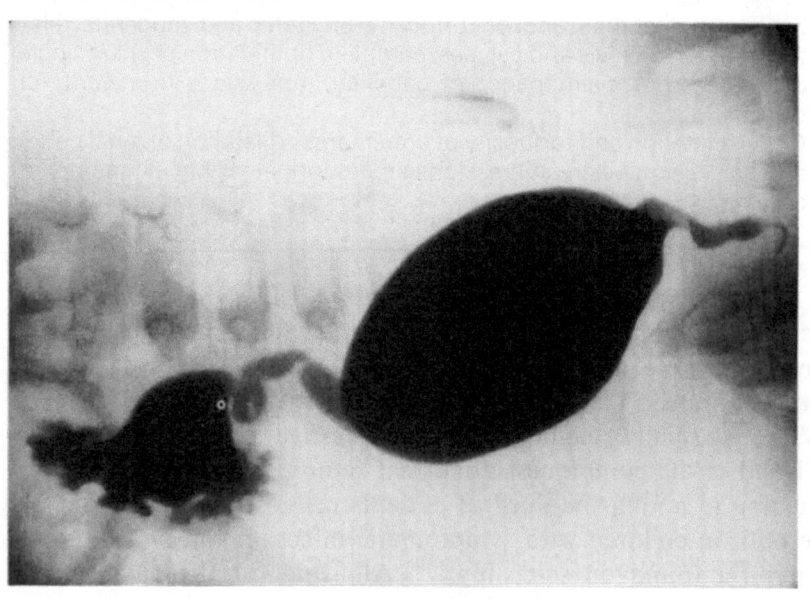

FIGURE 2.2 (a) MCU in 3-month-old male infant following UTI. Fetal urinary tract dilatation suspected on antenatal ultrasonography at 20 and 24 weeks. Postnatal ultrasound at 6 days reported to be normal. (b) IVU at 4 months in same infant

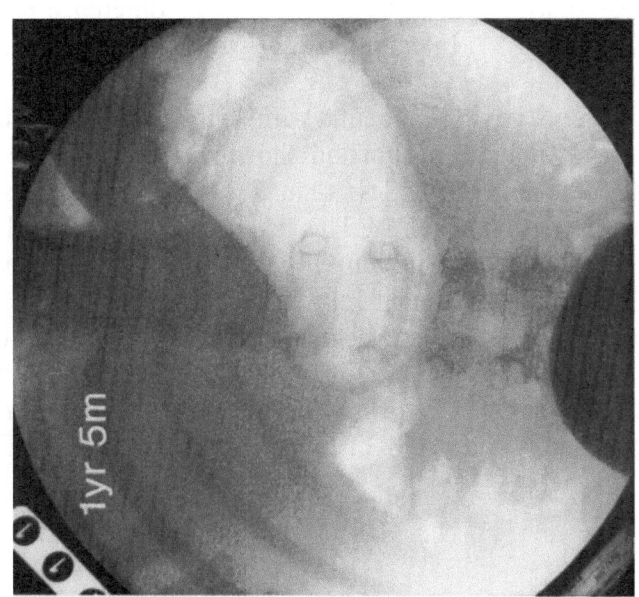

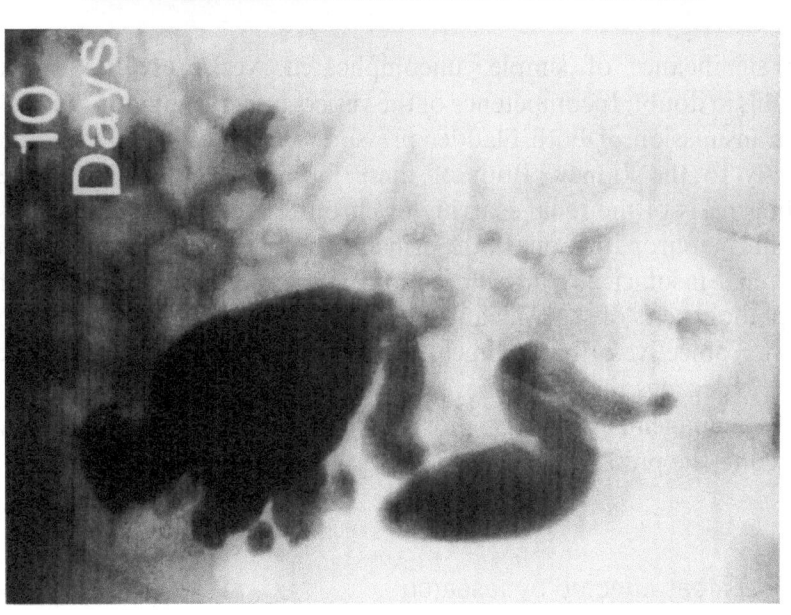

FIGURE 2.3   Contrast cystograms at (a) 10 days and (b) 1 year 5 months in infant boy showing spontaneous disappearance of vesico-ureteric reflux. He was maintained on low-dose antibacterial prophylaxis

schoolgirls, a much lower proportion of the black girls had VUR when compared with the white girls[17] and this difference has been confirmed by others[19,20]. Infection as a possible aetiological factor is discussed later.

Baker *et al.*[21], studying patients with 'infravesical obstruction' and UTI, noted that the proportion showing VUR decreased with age from 60% in infancy to less than 7% in adults, suggesting a spontaneous resolution of reflux. This has been shown to be the case in prospective studies of children with urinary infection in several countries[2,3,5,22–26]. Improvement or disappearance is more likely to take place with less severe degrees of reflux. Only 30–40% of Grades IV or V reflux (IRSC grading) might be expected to disappear (due probably to greater deformity of the vesico-ureteric junction) compared with more than 80% of the less severe grades (see Figures 2.3a and b).

Significance

The significance of simple, uncomplicated, vesico-ureteric reflux remains in doubt. Incompetence of the vesico-ureteric junction permits the transmission of both bladder pressure and any bladder bacteria directly to the kidney. Both of these factors are involved in the pathogenesis of the renal scarring of chronic atrophic pyelonephritis or reflux nephropathy, one of the principal causes of both hypertension and renal insufficiency in children and young adults. Elucidation of the pathogenesis of scarring and its limitation or prevention has been a major objective of both clinical and experimental research over the last two decades.

The management and prognosis of the child with UTI is closely related to the presence or absence of vesico-ureteric reflux.

Clinical areas affected by research

Much attention was paid in the 1950's to 'chronic pyelonephritis' and its relationship to hypertension[27]. In the early 1960's, observations on its association with VUR by Hodson and Edwards[28] and Hutch and colleagues[29] focused attention on reflux and corrective operations were therefore devised. These were not always successful, and, after observing the ill-effects on the kidney of occasional postoperative vesico-ureteric junction obstruction, we set about exploring whether reflux alone without infection was damaging to the kidney. We used a regimen of low-dose antibacterial prophylaxis, regular bladder emptying and double micturition which was very effective in preventing recurrent infection[30]. Not only did the kidneys grow satisfactorily without further scarring, but all except the most severe reflux tended to resolve spontaneously with time[31].

Over the past decade, research has continued into various aspects of VUR. Those principally affecting clinical practice include the aetiology of VUR and improved methods of diagnosis and investigation, the effect of VUR with and without UTI and the most appropriate management of patients with VUR.

It is increasingly evident that it is in infancy and childhood that the effect of VUR is particularly important. Hence, this chapter will mainly deal with VUR in this age group.

AETIOLOGY

Primary reflux

Most VUR is congenital or 'primary' and may be associated with laterally displaced incompetent ureteric orifices, or with paraureteric diverticula or ectopic ureters, or with other renal anomalies, such as duplex, dysplastic or horseshoe kidneys. There may be a short intramural segment of the ureter, perhaps due to delayed 'maturation' of the vesico-ureteric junction or to a deficiency of the muscle of the tunnel roof[24]. VUR has also been classified on the basis of the cystoscopic appearances: that is, on the position and configuration of the orifice[32] and on the length of the intramural ureter[25]. However, cystoscopic appearances are observer dependent and will also vary with the volume of fluid introduced into the bladder at cystoscopy or with the intravesical pressure. Apart from those with grossly abnormal ureteric orifices (golf-hole) and large paraureteric diverticula, Brock and Kaplan did not find the endoscopic appearance helpful in predicting which patients would spontaneously stop refluxing[33]. Furthermore, Duckett and Bellinger[34] showed that, unless the ureteric orifices were grossly abnormal, there was only a 50% correlation between their appearances and the likelihood of spontaneous cessation of reflux. Vermillion and Heale[35], studying 67 adult patients with 97 scarred kidneys, found on cystoscopy that, although 90% of the corresponding ureteric orifices were abnormal, only 46% of these continued to have demonstrable reflux on cystography.

Practical implications: Abnormal endoscopic appearances of the ureteric orifice may persist after reflux has ceased and, except when grossly abnormal, are not a reliable prognostic index. Cystoscopy is commonly performed as part of the preoperative evaluation of the patient, although not as part of the routine investigation of the child with UTI or VUR.

Genetics and family studies

VUR has been reported in identical twins[36] and in triplets[37] and surveys have indicated that there is a genetic predisposition to VUR in some families[38]. The mode of inheritance of reflux is unclear, some authors suggesting that this may be multifactorial, with functional expression at the vesico-ureteric junction dependent on a variety of environmental factors[39], while others postulate autosomal dominant inheritance with variable penetrance[40]. There is a male preponderance in some families. There are a number of family studies, including those of Bailey in New Zealand[40], who found a 34% overall incidence of VUR in 88 families of refluxing children (27% of siblings, 13% of offspring and 14% of parents); Atwell *et al.* in Britain who found 20 siblings and 9 parents of 35 children with VUR to have either reflux or a bifid renal pelvis[41]; and Goldraich *et al.* who investigated 51 parents and 43 siblings of 26 Brazilian children with primary reflux and found VUR or reflux nephropathy in 70% overall, 23% of siblings and 12% of parents[42]. Jerkins and Noe screened 104 siblings of 78 index patients with reflux and found 34 to have reflux: 25 of these were symptomless and uninfected[43]. The incidence of VUR was higher in the siblings of index patients who had renal scarring in addition to VUR. In the families of 89 index patients among those with VUR under our care, reflux has been demonstrated in 34 of 74 siblings and 3 of 24 offspring investigated. Eight parents have severe reflux nephropathy.

Chapmen *et al.*[44] have recently reported a complex segregation analysis applied to data from 88 families in which at least one member had VUR. Their results support their view of an autosomal dominant inheritance, and indicate that close relatives of patients with RN and VUR should be investigated.

Practical clinical implications: It is generally recommended that infants born to parents known to have VUR or whose siblings are known to have VUR should be screened for reflux during the neonatal period. It may be possible to identify a dilated urinary tract by ultrasound, although a normal result will not necessarily exclude VUR. VUR may also be suspected on an antenatal ultrasound scan.

Other siblings of index patients with severe VUR or reflux nephropathy should also be investigated.

Secondary or acquired reflux

Vesico-ureteric reflux may develop:

1. Following calculous or other traumatic damage to the vesico-ureteric junction;
2. As a result of impaired neurological control of bladder function because of trauma, surgery, or a neural tube defect;
3. In association with dysfunctional voiding; or
4. Secondary to mechanical obstruction, such as posterior urethral valves or ureterocoele.

Urodynamics

The more refined techniques of studying bladder function originally applied to children with known neurological abnormalities, such as spinal dysraphism, have been particularly important, both in terms of defining normal bladder function and in establishing the relationship between bladder voiding pressures, vesico-ureteric reflux, ureteric function and their effect on the kidney[45,46]. It is well known that, in children with neuropathic bladder, secondary reflux may develop within a few years. Woods and Atwell[47] studied 96 children with spinal dysraphism and found reflux in 28% at one year and 45% at five years. It is now suggested that some VUR previously thought to be congenital is secondary to detrusor sphincter dyssynergia. Bauer *et al.*[48] found VUR in 50% of children with 'non-neurogenic neurogenic bladder' and Van Gool *et al.* in 4% of children with detrusor sphincter dyssynergia[46]. Taylor *et al.*[49] demonstrated bladder instability in 28 (75%) of 37 girls with VUR; this correlated closely with symptoms of urge incontinence, frequency and nocturnal enuresis. Furthermore, in patients with neuropathic bladder, the risk of renal damage is greater in those with high-pressure voiding and reflux than in those with low-pressure reflux[46].

Clinical applications: Attention to the details of bladder function and voiding pattern are an important part of the clinical history of children with VUR and also of those with UTI. Management is considered in a later section.

DIAGNOSIS

VUR causes few symptoms other than those due to associated urinary infection, hypertension or renal insufficiency. It may, however, cause loin pain during micturition, particularly after either a long interval without voiding or a large drink, or with high pressure voiding due to impaired outflow. It may be suspected when there is a significant post-micturition residue, either clinically on double micturition (i.e. when voiding is repeated after 2–5 minutes), or on IVU or ultrasound. This is due to the return to the bladder of refluxed urine after micturition.

Imaging

Ultrasound

The diagnosis may be suspected when the renal pelvis or ureter is noted to be dilated on ultrasonography when the bladder is full, or if the bladder remains filled following micturition. While ultra-sonography has the advantage of being non-invasive and free from radiation, it is relatively insensitive and reflux cannot be excluded by a negative scan[50]. It may also miss associated renal abnormalities, such as duplex, renal scarring and evidence of renal inflammation.

The antenatal appearance of fetal pelviureteric dilatation, though sometimes considered to be 'physiological', may be due to VUR and thus an important marker for detecting VUR before infection and renal damage has supervened[52,53].

Until the significance of such dilatation of the fetal urinary tract (which may be intermittent) is better understood, it is essential that obstetricians, ultrasonographers, paediatricians and paediatric sur-geons collect and document this information. Infants in whom dila-tation has been seen should be followed carefully beyond the postnatal period.

A postnatal ultrasound scan will usually detect obstruction. If, however, the infant is poorly hydrated or has an empty bladder, it may fail to demonstrate ureteric dilatation associated with reflux. Infants with VUR may thus subsequently present with a urinary infection.

Practical clinical implications: Thomas recommends performing cystography in infants in whom minor antenatal dilatation has been found. If this is normal, he suggests[51] repeating the ultrasound scan at three months of age. (Figures 2.2a and b).

An increased ureteric calibre on IVU may suggest that VUR is present, although this sign may persist after reflux has ceased and may not be obvious if the IVU is carried out in a poorly hydrated patient. Stri-ations of the renal pelvis may also be seen.

Contrast micturating cystourethrography

The contrast radiographic cystourethrogram remains at present the definitive method for diagnosing reflux. In both boys and girls, it is desirable to make or confirm the initial diagnosis in this way in order to visualize the morphology of the bladder and ureter and to assess the urethral calibre[54].

The cystogram should be carried out in a wakeful child and reflux is sought during both filling and voiding phases and the bladder neck and urethra observed. The bladder residual urine, capacity and function can be assessed, morphological abnormalities, such as diverticula and ureterocoele, seen and intrarenal reflux (IRR) or urethral calibre variation, particularly in the male, detected. Furthermore, a visual image is obtained which simplifies explanation to the parents and the child, and thus increases their compliance in management. The prognosis is closely related to the severity of reflux based upon radiological appearances and this is a better guide than cystoscopy[34]. In most infants and children, the MCU will follow a urinary infection (deferred for at least two weeks to allow any bladder mucosal inflammation to subside); thus, they will usually be receiving low-dose antibacterial prophylaxis. If not, the procedure should be covered by a three-day umbrella of a suitable antibacterial drug, such as trimethoprim, co-trimoxazole or nitrofurantoin. The cystogram will be completed more rapidly and effectively if the parents and child are well informed about the procedure and the child's confidence and cooperation gained. It should be carried out by those with experience with children.

However, contrast voiding cystography has several disadvantages. Passage of even a fine polythene catheter can cause discomfort. In infant boys with possible posterior urethral valves, experience in catheterization is essential to avoid damage to the urethra. If urethral narrowing or stenosis is suspected, contrast can be introduced suprapubically. Some gonadal radiation exposure is inevitable, though this should be minimized by careful preparation of the child and supervision by an experienced radiologist.

Various non-invasive diagnostic methods have been explored, such as examining the urine for N-acetylglucosaminidase (NAG), Tamm Horsfall or other proteins, without any consistent correlation being found with VUR. The advent of nuclear medicine offered the possibility of reducing radiation exposure[55].

Radionuclide cystography

Indirect radionuclide cystography

This has the advantage of not involving catheterization. It depends upon the rapid clearance through the glomeruli of a labelled isotope, usually ^{99m}Tc diethylenetriaminepenta-acetic acid (DTPA) injected intravenously. An increase in the radioactivity in the renal areas during and after micturition usually indicates VUR. There are, however, disadvantages in this method. First, since the child must be able to void on request, it cannot be used in infancy or those not yet toilet trained. Second, it is affected both by the renal function and by the state of hydration of the patient and by delay in flow at the pelviureteric junction. Slow clearance of isotope, resulting in high background levels will obscure minor degrees of reflux and make interpretation difficult. Reflux is detected by this method mainly during and after voiding, so that minor degrees of low-pressure reflux may be missed. Conway considers that up to 25% of reflux may be missed on indirect radionuclide cystography[56]. A recent comparison of indirect radionuclide cystography using DTPA with contrast cystography in a group of 47 children aged 5–15 years showed good agreement in only 61% of potentially refluxing renal units, though there was overall agreement in 88% of those with severe reflux[57]. There is probably little difference in radiation exposure between the indirect radionuclide cystogram (when voiding may be delayed for some time) and the carefully performed contrast cystogram[55].

Practical implications: In view of these limitations emerging from careful comparisons with other methods, the value of indirect radionuclide cystography (IRNC) is somewhat restricted. Unnecessary catheterization can be avoided by its use in girls over the age of 5, in the medical follow up of children with reflux and can also be combined with a DTPA renogram in the postoperative investigation of children undergoing ureteric re-implantation.

Direct radionuclide cystography

This is considered to be a more sensitive method of detecting VUR. It delivers significantly less radiation than the formal contrast cystogram but does involve catheterization. Good quantitative information about bladder function is provided[56]. Further refinements of this method are likely to lead to greater sensitivity in the detection of minor degrees of reflux. Its use has also been suggested in the investigation of siblings of patients with reflux or with renal scarring[58]. As with contrast cystography, a suprapublic approach can be used.

Practical implications: It appears that, although ultrasound may demonstrate urinary tract dilatation and indirect nuclear cystography may reliably indicate severe VUR, negative findings do not exclude its presence. Contrast cystography at present remains the initial diagnostic method of choice, providing anatomical details of the kidney, bladder and urethra which are essential in the evaluation of the child's urinary tract. Direct radionuclide cystography appears to be equally reliable in follow-up studies. Both involve catheterization, but contrast or isotope can be introduced suprapubically if urethral stenosis is suspected.

ASSESSMENT AND FURTHER INVESTIGATION OF THE PATIENT WITH REFLUX

The assessment of a child with VUR includes the past and present history of urinary tract infection, of voiding patterns and bowel habits and also a family history of renal or bladder problems or of hypertension. Measurement of the child's blood pressure, height and weight, urine microscopy, culture and routine testing and determination of the renal morphology and function, form the baseline upon which management is planned, and its success evaluated. Good renal growth without the development of new renal scars is the objective.

The initial IVU

This gives an estimate of renal size, shape, function and parenchymal thickness with which subsequent standard films can be compared.

Claësson *et al.* have extended Hodson's early charts relating renal length to height so that interpolar length and various measurements of parenchymal thickness can be related to the height of a lumbar vertebra[59]. If there has been a recent infection, there may be local or general swelling and a reduced nephrogram. The classical radiological signs of renal scarring are well established and include coarse irregularly distributed scars with thinned parenchyma overlying distorted or clubbed calyces, most commonly seen at upper or lower poles. If they are not distributed generally, there may be intervening normal renal segments which will hypertrophy.

Radionuclide renography

Merrick *et al.*[60], using ^{99m}Tc dimercaptosuccinic acid (DMSA), demonstrated that areas of defective isotope uptake, due to locally impaired renal function, correlated well with radiological renal scars. In some, there was simply a reduction in total renal function. Although non-specific, these appearances are seen particularly in patients with reflux nephropathy. More widespread patchy impairment of function has been demonstrated on DMSA scanning during or immediately after urinary tract infection in children with VUR[61]. These photon-deficient areas can be reversible and can disappear after treatment of an acute infection and should not be termed 'scars'. Further comparisons between the IVU and the DMSA have been carried out in patients with VUR with satisfactory correlation between the findings[42,62]. It is generally felt that the two investigations are complementary, the IVU providing morphological and the DMSA providing functional information, including the proportion of function contributed by each kidney (Figure 2.4).

Ultrasound

Experience of this technique is being gained rapidly but it remains observer dependent and subjective. With more parallel evaluation against established methods and wider experience and expertise, it should become increasingly useful. It is helpful in identifying

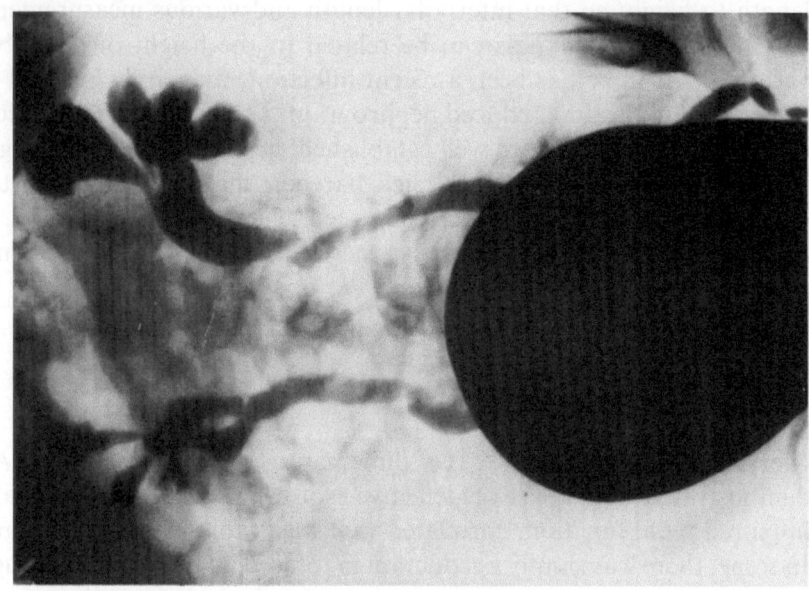

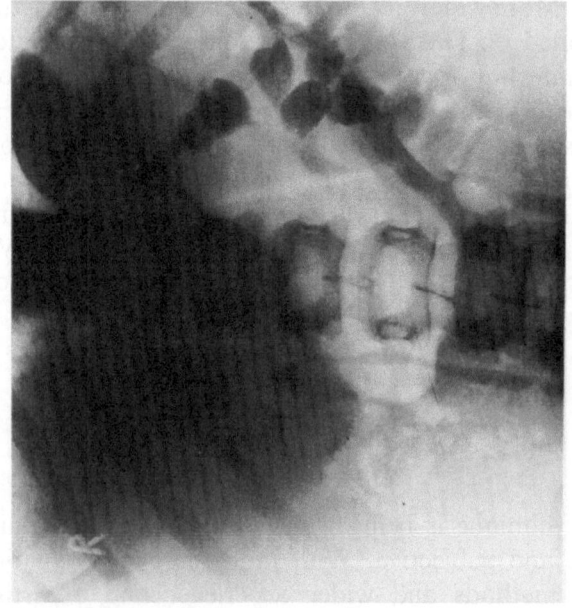

FIGURE 2.4 (a) IVU

(b) MCU

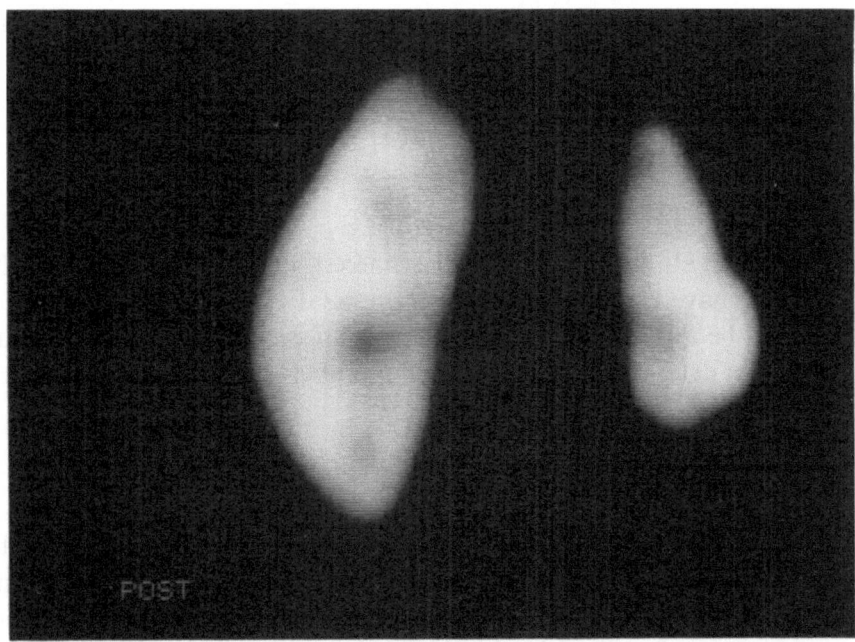

FIGURE 2.4 (c) DMSA scan (posterior view) in a girl aged 5 with previous history of recurrent UTI. There is a bilateral severe reflux (b) and bilateral renal scarring (a). The smaller right kidney (c) with irregular contour contributes only 31% of the total function, the left kidney showing calyceal dilatation and impaired isotope uptake in the upper pole, 69%

pelviureteric dilatation or significantly reduced or increased renal size, without necessarily identifying renal scars, duplex kidneys or infected renal involvement in a child with VUR and UTI[51].

Urodynamics

A careful voiding history is essential, since this has been shown to correlate with urodynamic findings[47]. When a neurological deficit is present or detrusor sphincter dyssynergia or an unstable bladder suspected from the history, pressure and flow studies or more complex urodynamic assessments can be combined with either voiding contrast cystourethrography or with direct radionuclide cystography.

Acute UTI

If the patient with VUR develops a symptomatic UTI with high fever, the ESR and C reactive protein have been shown to relate well to other evidence of renal involvement.

Renal function

Plasma creatinine is the usual baseline estimate of renal function. If patients have evidence of renal damage, a GFR or creatinine clearance should be estimated together with an assessment of individual renal function determined by isotope renography.

Proteinuria

The work of Kincaid Smith and Becker has shown that, in patients with reflux nephropathy, especially if accompanied by hypertension, diffuse parenchymal lesions, including periglomerular fibrosis and tubular atrophy, may develop[63]. This is seen particularly in the older patient and is accompanied by proteinuria. They have also shown that marked proteinuria is a poor prognostic sign in these patients and may be the forerunner of rapid irreversible deterioration in renal function[64].

Somatic growth

There have been few satisfactory reports of somatic growth following surgical correction of reflux. However, in 38 girls receiving co-tri-moxazole prophylaxis, normal growth in height was seen during two to four years of persisting sterile reflux[65].

Follow up

This involves careful monitoring of urinary tract infection, somatic growth and blood pressure with assessment of proteinuria and renal function if there is any renal damage. Satisfactory renal growth without scarring on a one-film IVU at 2–3-year intervals (after one year in infancy) is more important than repeating the cystogram. This may only be necessary to confirm cessation of reflux or as a preoperative measure if it has not been possible to control recurrent infection.

THE EFFECT OF VUR WITH AND WITHOUT UTI

Much controversy has centred on the effect of reflux on the kidney. Can renal damage, such as focal scarring and generally thinned parenchyma, be caused by reflux alone, or is obstruction or infection also necessary? Indeed, can renal scarring occur without reflux?

These matters are of some practical importance, since approximately a quarter of all the children and young adults entering the European dialysis and transplant programme have renal failure due to reflux nephropathy (RN) or chronic atrophic pyelonephritis[66]. 10–25% of patients with RN will develop hypertension within ten years, even if their VUR has been corrected surgically. The risk is greater if renal scarring is bilateral but hypertension can develop even in patients with unilateral scarring[67,68].

Much of the recent research into reflux nephropathy is collected in two volumes, each jointly edited by Hodson[69,70].

The effect of reflux and pressure: sterile reflux

Clinical observations

In 1969, Hutch and Smith[71] published a series of 24 patients with sterile reflux. Twenty-three were young male adults and showed uniform parenchymal thinning with hydronephrosis but no renal scars; it is likely that there was some outflow obstruction with high-pressure reflux but this is not mentioned. Studies of renal function in children with VUR before and after its surgical correction[72] and of renal growth following surgery have suggested that severe reflux at least has a damaging effect on the kidney. In some reports, however, the precise relationship of the studies to the timing of the preceding infection is not clear, and Aperia et al.[73] have indicated that, although they found impaired renal function in their patients with VUR, they also noted that this was closely related to infection and improved when infection was treated[74].

Urodynamic studies in patients with neuropathic bladder have indicated that those with VUR and high bladder pressures have the greatest risk of deterioration of renal function[75]. Even more susceptible are those in whom UTI is superimposed on high-pressure VUR[47].

In a series of 201 children with 302 refluxing ureters, maintained on long-term low-dose prophylaxis[76], 214 refluxing renal units remained free from infection over 2–12 years' observation. No new scars developed and renal growth continued within one standard deviation of that expected in 213 kidneys, even in 21 renal units with scarring on entry and 30 with severe reflux.

Opportunities to make further closely monitored clinical assessments of the effect of sterile reflux are provided by the child with the neuropathic bladder and by the symptomless uninfected infant or sibling with no past history of urinary infection found on screening investigation to have VUR.

Experimental studies

Hodson et al. used a piglet model which has a multipapillary kidney similar to the human and in which intrarenal reflux can occur. Reflux was induced unilaterally and the urethra was partially obstructed in order to produce high-pressure VUR. They noted the development of renal scars without introducing infection; that is, scars due to sterile high-pressure reflux[77]. This occurred only in piglets with partial urethral obstruction and intravesical pressures of more than 45 cm H_2O. Ransley and Risden were unable to reproduce Hobson's results with sterile reflux in piglets with lower bladder pressures[78]. In a more recent extension of their studies, they found that a combination of high voiding pressure and elevated resting pressures over a prolonged period did result in the formation of renal scars in piglets with sterile urine[79]. Furthermore, they examined the effect of high- and low-pressure sterile reflux in a growing one-kidney minipig model. Over a period of five months, there was no effect on GFR or on renal growth, but there was a significant reduction in the renal concentrating capacity[80].

Experimental evidence does, therefore, suggest that scarring secondary to sterile reflux can occur, although probably only in association with extreme urological dysfunction.

Clinical application: High-pressure reflux associated with any degree of outflow obstruction may cause damage to the kidneys like obstructive atrophy. Clinically, this is an uncommon situation and is likely to occur only with abnormalities such as posterior urethral valves or a severely hypertonic neuropathic bladder. Increasingly infants with congenital obstructive lesions should be recognized by antenatal ultrasound.

Vesico-ureteric reflux and urinary tract infection

Clinical observations

Reflux is most commonly diagnosed during the investigation of childhood UTI and the two are clearly closely associated. It has been postulated that infection may cause VUR but there is no good experimental evidence to support this. Where the intramural ureter is short and the vesico-ureteric valve barely competent, the oedema of acute cystitis could stiffen the orifice and cause VUR. Cystograms are not intentionally performed during an infection and no evidence has yet emerged from other techniques to support this theory. In some series, the percentage of bacteriuric children with reflux has decreased with age, suggesting that a developmental anomaly of the vesico-ureteric junction is the main cause of VUR, while, in others, no significant change in incidence has been observed.

On the other hand, does reflux predispose to urinary tract infection? Evidence both in favour of and against this idea has been presented, though, on theoretical grounds, any condition which results in stasis of residual urine within the bladder could increase the risk of bacterial infection[81].

Follow up of a cohort of schoolgirls with covert bacteriuria in the Cardiff–Oxford study showed no significant difference in persistence or recurrence of bacteriuria between those with and those without

VUR. There is, however, evidence that VUR facilitates the passage of infection to the kidney. Comparison of the presenting symptoms of UTI in 744 children with and without reflux showed that fever was twice as common in those with reflux as in those without, suggesting renal involvement[14]. Preliminary results of the International Reflux Study have shown no difference in recurrence rates of infection between medical and surgical groups in the six months before and after surgery, but significantly fewer 'pyelonephritic' episodes after reflux has stopped[82]. Elo *et al.* reported a similar experience[83].

Of some importance is the proportion of children with VUR and/or UTI who have scarred kidneys. Severe reflux can be associated with renal dysplasia; although the kidneys may be abnormal from birth, further renal scarring can result from UTI. The figure for renal scarring among children with UTI rises steadily with age, recurrence of infection[84] and duration of symptoms. For children with VUR, the proportion with renal scarring also rises with age. Among 331 refluxing renal units, Smellie *et al.* found the proportion with scarred kidneys increased from 12.5% of those presenting aged 2, through 40% for 7–9-year-olds, to 63% for those between 11 and 13 years of age[85]. These observations indicate that renal scars may be acquired and that, not only VUR, but also UTI is needed for renal scarring to develop.

We found further evidence for this in a series of 201 children with 302 refluxing units maintained on a medical regimen[76]. Eighty-eight refluxing units, 24 with renal scarring, were exposed to breakthrough infection, 81 of them single episodes. Unlike the 214 units which remained uninfected and grew well, renal growth was slowed in 16 of these kidneys, 10 of them already scarred. In two kidneys, new scars developed, one in a previously normal and one in an already scarred kidney, both following symptomatic infection. Most of the 16 renal units in which progress was unsatisfactory had gross reflux and extensive established renal scarring, a situation which is least likely to respond well to any form of therapy.

Experimental evidence

Hodson *et al.,* using the piglet model, demonstrated the development of scarring similar to human chronic atrophic pyelonephritis after inducing reflux and introducing infection to the bladder[77].

Ransley and Risden, in another series of experiments using a similar piglet model with unilateral reflux, were able to produce classical coarse renal scarring of the kidney drained by the refluxing ureter after introducing infection into the bladder. The scars developed in compound papillae. No scarring developed in the opposite non-refluxing ureter. Furthermore, no scarring developed in the kidney with or without VUR when the urinary tract was kept sterile by low-dose antibacterial prophylaxis[78].

They suggested that maximal infective renal damage may occur with the first UTI in a child with VUR and that the distribution of the scarring is predetermined by the renal morphology and disposition of compound papillae. This would explain why some children with VUR and UTI never develop scars, and why most scarring develops early in childhood and is located mainly at the poles, the most common site for compound papillae in the human. Distortion of adjacent papillae and their duct orifices by contracting scars could allow new scars to develop at a later date.

Particularly important was their extension of this work to study the effect of therapy. In the same model, they showed that, if full-dose antibacterial treatment of the piglet was started within 4–5 days of introducing infection to the bladder, renal scarring was modified or even prevented[86] (see Figure 2.5). Similar results were reported by Miller and Phillips using a rat model[88].

Acquired renal scars

Clinical evidence

The limited documentation of acquired renal scars, i.e. scars developing in previously normal kidneys or in new areas of previously scarred kidneys, has been variously attributed:

1. Scars may all represent congenital areas of dysplasia;
2. They may develop in early infancy and childhood when a urinary infection may not be recognized;
3. They may follow the first UTI which, in girls, is not always routinely investigated, and an IVU may appear normal, so that scarring is already established when investigation follows a second or third UTI.

Furthermore, established scarring is permanent, whereas VUR may cease, and adults with a scarred kidney may have neither VUR nor a recognized history of UTI.

Hypoplasia and dysplasia can undoubtedly be linked with VUR, particularly the most severe grades, but children reported to have developed new scars in previously normal kidneys probably represent the tip of the iceberg of the majority of patients with scarred kidneys. Their initial 'normal' IVU following a UTI may show minor changes, such as swelling or a locally reduced nephrogram, which is only seen as a scar when, for some reason, the IVU is repeated at a later date.

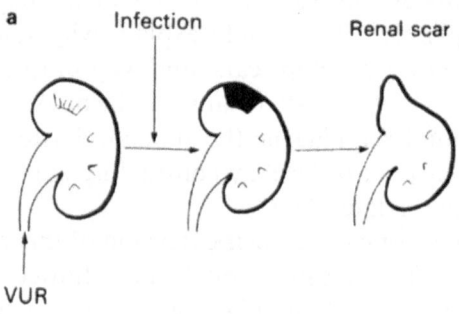

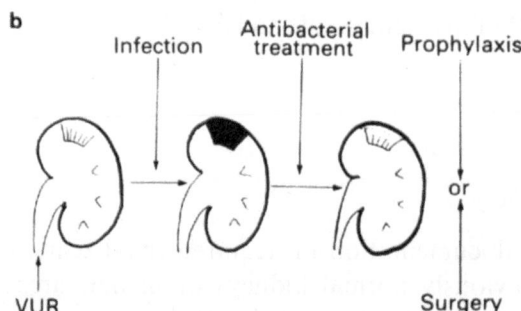

FIGURE 2.5   Diagrammatic representation of:
(a) New scar development (after Ransley and Risdon[78])
(b) Experimental prevention or modification of new renal scarring by rapid introduction of antibacterial therapy[86].
[Reproduced from Smellie, J. M. and Normand, I. C. S. (1985). Urinary tract infection 1985. *Postgrad. Med. J.*, **61**, 895–905 (p. 902), with permission of Macmillan Press Ltd.[87]]

(The interval between the initial IVU and the first showing renal scarring does not necessarily indicate the time taken for scarring to develop.) The DMSA scan on which areas of defective isotope uptake may be seen, both during the immediate inflammatory stage after infection and also at a later date when a classical scar is discernible on the IVU, will be valuable in elucidating the natural history of renal scarring.

Some features were shared by almost all of the 300 or so patients with acquired renal scars well documented in the literature. They were children aged 12 or less, many of them under 5, and had symptomatic infection of a refluxing urinary tract[68].

Infection has almost invariably occurred in children developing new scars. Winberg *et al.* have emphasized the susceptibility of the young growing kidney to infective damage[89] and most of the infants and children seen with reflux nephropathy will present with already established scarring, possibly because the process is more rapid in infancy, perhaps because a urinary infection causing only fever and non-specific symptoms is often overlooked. The Swedish group also pointed out the serious effects of persistent untreated infection and, in recent studies of children developing new scars, delay in starting effective treatment has been a marked feature[90,91]. Among 74 such children collected from a number of centres, over half of the ill children waited for four or more days before effective antibacterial treatment was started, and nearly half of those with low-grade symptoms waited for up to three months[91]. In the same study, it was shown that the development of new scars is not confined to the preschool age group, and, based upon the child's age at the last 'normal' IVU, at least a third of the 74 children developing scarring had normal kidneys at five, and in 38 kidneys (44%), scars developed at five years or over. New scars developed in 18 kidneys which were already scarred, 9 of them over the age of five (Figure 2.6).

Frequently recurring urinary infection was another characteristic feature. All the children who developed new scars in previously scarred kidneys had a recurrence of symptomatic infection, also noted by others[4,92], and none receiving uninterrupted prophylaxis.

Finally, in Smellie's collaborative study, VUR was seen in 67 of the 74 children developing new scars and in all but one of those who had a technically satisfactory cystogram immediately after presentation.

Reflux was only mild to moderate in 36 kidneys, but, in general, the more extensive new scarring developed where reflux was most severe[91].

Similar findings were reported by Winter et al.[90], namely symptomatic infection preceding scar development; there was often delay

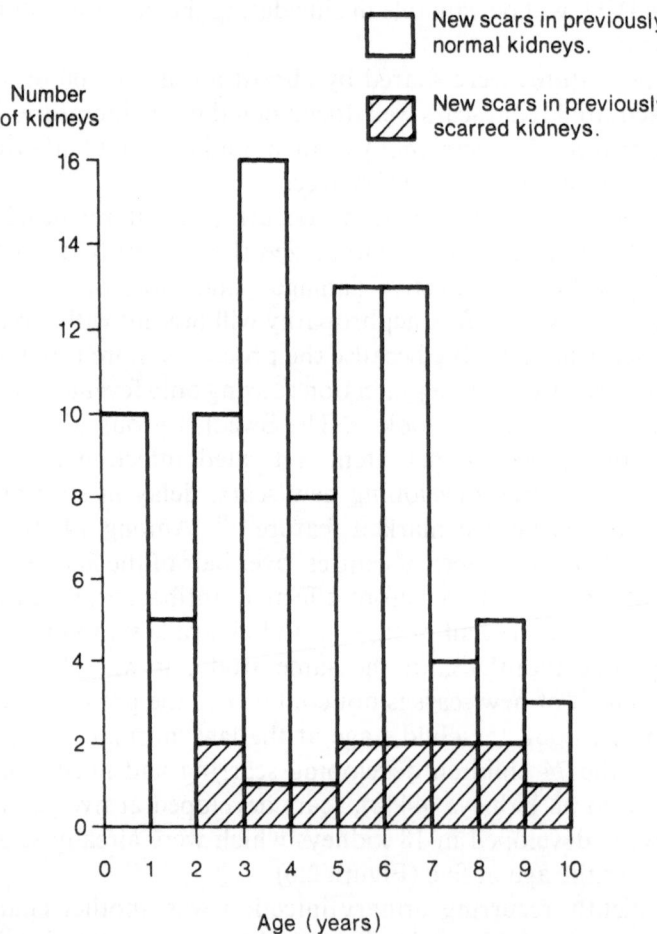

FIGURE 2.6 Age at which new renal scars appeared in 87 kidneys among 74 children[91]. The age of the child indicates when the IVU was last normal or unscarred in a segment subsequently showing scarring. There was wide variation in the interval between this and the subsequent IVU showing new scarring so that scars were often first recognized in much older children

in the start of effective treatment; infection recurred and scarring was less severe when prophylaxis had been used; but, unlike other accounts, only half the ureters had demonstrable reflux[90].

Social problems, such as family illness, stress from parental separation and frequent rehousing, are important in interfering with compliance and continuity of care. Undoubtedly some of these children have suffered 'social scarring'.

Covert bacteriuria: In the Cardiff–Oxford Study, no new scars developed in initially normal kidneys on follow up of children with VUR and continuing asymptomatic bacteriuria. In half of the girls who had renal scarring in addition to reflux and bacteriuria, further scars developed in previously normal areas[18].

Intrarenal reflux: Rolleston *et al.* noted that, in infants, new scars tended to develop in renal segments where intrarenal reflux (IRR) or calyco-tubular backflow had previously been visualized[3].

Ransley and Risden, studying the renal papillary morphology, showed that simple conical renal papillae with slit-like duct orifices do not permit IRR, whereas compound renal papillae, most commonly situated at the renal poles and found in approximately 75% of humans, allow IRR into the centrally placed collecting ducts with open orifices[93]. This has been confirmed by Tamminen and others in autopsy material[94,95].

Clinical application: It appears from clinical and experimental observations that the reflux of infected urine at normal voiding pressure up to a kidney with compound papillae in a growing child is the major cause of new renal scars developing, and that treatment should be aimed at preventing infection or stopping reflux[96].

MANAGEMENT

The principal aims of management of children with VUR are:

1. The detection of VUR and documentation of the presence or absence of renal scars;

2. The rapid treatment of clinical acute pyelonephritis and the prevention of further symptomatic infection;
3. The prevention of further new renal scarring; and
4. The promotion of normal renal and somatic growth.

Long-term follow up of the child with established renal scarring is essential in order to detect complications, such as hypertension and impaired renal function, at an early stage.

Acute infection

Clinical and experimental evidence has indicated that rapid effective antibacterial treatment of UTI associated with VUR can limit, or possibly prevent, the development of renal scarring. Thus, particularly in infants and young children who are at the greatest risk of developing scars, appropriate antibiotics should be commenced as soon as any infection is suspected. The antibacterial regimen can be modified when the results of the urine culture are available or if there is no clinical response within 48 hours. Five days of full-dose treatment is usually given for first infections, when the underlying pathology is unknown, and for those with known VUR. This can then be followed immediately by a low dose of a suitable antibacterial drug until investigation of the urinary tract has been completed, thus preventing rapid reinfection of the susceptible renal tract.

Investigation

The methods of diagnosing VUR, their advantages and disadvantages have already been discussed. Until alternative techniques have been further refined and comparison made, contrast cystography will remain the baseline investigation to establish bladder and urethral anatomy and function, to assess reflux severity and detect paraureteric diverticula and IRR. The IVU and DMSA are complementary in assessing the upper renal tract.

Ultrasound will highlight severe abnormalities but will not recognize inflammatory change, is unreliable in detecting scars and, particularly for growth assessment, is dependent upon the experience, skill and continuity of the ultrasonographer.

All the investigative methods should be tailored to the patient's needs and both irradiation and discomfort minimized. Local practice will vary according to the equipment, experience and expertise available.

Medical management of children with VUR

The purpose of medical management is to prevent recurrent infection and to reduce back-pressure effects while the vesico-ureteric valve remains incompetent.

Lenaghan et al.[92], using double micturition and intermittent short courses of antibacterial treatment for recurrent symptomatic infection in 102 children with VUR, observed resolution of reflux in 26% of dilated ureters and 66% of those with milder reflux, but new scars were seen in 16 of 76 kidneys thought initially to be normal. (In a footnote to their paper, the authors comment that had prophylaxis been available when they started the study, recurrent infections and renal scarring might have been reduced.)

The alternative and more effective regimen of medical management is to reinforce the natural defence mechanisms which reduce the risk of bacterial colonization of the bladder and combine this with uninterrupted low-dose antibacterial prophylaxis[97-99]. Thus, in infants and young children, an adequate fluid intake, especially in hot weather, and attention to bowel function are recommended. In the toilet-trained child, a routine may be established of regular but not excessive drinks, regular frequent complete voiding at intervals of 2–3 hours, double micturition at bedtime and a daily motion.

To cover this programme, particularly while the tissues of the kidney and urinary tract are recovering from recent inflammation, low-dose antibacterial prophylaxis is given. This treatment has usually been continued while VUR is present or until after puberty. The appropriate duration is currently being studied. However, since it is known that significant renal scars can still develop in later childhood[91], it is advisable to continue so long as reflux extending up to the kidney persists.

67

Progress is monitored:

1. By urine culture at regular intervals and if the patient is febrile or unwell, and
2. By assessing renal growth and function.

If renal growth is satisfactory, follow-up cystography can be postponed until there is no residue on double micturition. The indirect isotope cystogram may give equivocal results and the other two methods involve catheterization.

Suitable drugs for prophylactic use should be excreted in high urinary concentration, effective against common urinary pathogens, should disturb faecal flora as little as possible and have a high margin of safety. They should be acceptable to the patient so that good compliance is achieved. The agents currently in regular use are nitrofurantoin, $1-2\,mg\,kg^{-1}\,day^{-1}$, or trimethoprim, $1-2\,mg\,kg^{-1}\,day^{-1}$, alone or in combination with sulphamethoxazole, $5-10\,mg\,kg^{-1}\,day^{-1}$, given in a single dose in the evening. Compliance will be improved by explaining the purpose of the prophylaxis to the parents and that the object is prevention and not therapy.

Recurrence of infection with an organism sensitive to the prophylactic drug suggests non-compliance or too low a dose; recurrence with a resistant organism indicates either too high a drug dose or persisting increased residual urine[84,101].

Using this regime, the UCH group have observed good control of infection[100,101] and normal renal growth[8], with the development of few scars and resolution of reflux in all but the most severe grades[97] and particularly in children with unilateral reflux[76]. The least satisfactory results were obtained in patients with gross reflux and established scarring. This experience has been shared by others[26,99,102].

Bladder instability

Homsy *et al.* have suggested that the use of the anticholinergic drug, oxybutynin, in children with VUR and detrusor sphincter dyssynergia increases the prospect of VUR cessation, but their study had no controls[103]. Koff and Murtagh, using anticholinergic drugs and antibacterial prophylaxis, found a reduced UTI recurrence rate and an increase in the rate of resolution of reflux compared with controls[104].

Their controls, however, were children with reflux but without evidence of disturbed bladder function. Taylor *et al.* found no difference in the rate of resolution of VUR in groups of children with stable or unstable severe reflux[49]. Older children with unstable bladders who would be likely to respond to specific treatment with anticholinergic drugs can usually be identified from their history. It has also been pointed out that the bladder training regimen for a child with an unstable bladder is similar to that used in the routine medical management of children with UTI and vesico-ureteric reflux[105].

In the infant and young child, current research would suggest that urodynamic studies should be undertaken if there is severe reflux since the effect of high-pressure reflux would be most deleterious in this age group.

Surgical management

Surgical correction by an experienced paediatric urologist offers a very good chance of 'cure' of VUR. A number of different procedures have been described, designed to increase the length of the submucosal ureteric tunnel in order to prevent VUR. Each technique has its advocates and all seem effective in experienced hands with success rates in reported series of between 95% and 98% in the short term[106,107]. Earlier reports included many children with mild reflux who would no longer be considered for surgical treatment. Coleman and McGovern, reviewing 20 years of reimplantation, reported 95.5% success in reimplanting 339 undilated refluxing ureters, compared with 22% initial success in 27 with dilated upper tracts and thickened bladder walls[108]. The less gratifying results of surgeons with less skill or experience are not usually published. The results of long-term follow up of patients undergoing the different techniques is needed, particularly through pregnancy, before a full evaluation can be made.

The most difficult patients to manage, surgically as well as medically, are those with atonic widely dilated ureters. These may result from the effect of infection on the ureter[109,110] or perhaps from prolonged exposure to high pressure as demonstrated by Jörgenson in the piglet[111]. Various tailoring procedures have been devised for reflux treatment in this group with success, but few reports are confined only

69

to the severely affected. Early complications of antireflux surgery are now uncommon in experienced hands. Ureterovesical stenosis or persistent reflux requiring further reimplantation, or reflux into the contralateral ureter have been reported in 3–5%[106].

In 1984, a new approach to the treatment of reflux was suggested. The periurethral injection of Teflon paste had been used successfully in the management of the elderly incontinent patient. O'Donnell and Puri showed, first in piglets and then in children, that a small endoscopic injection of polytef paste under the submucosal ureter produced a small encapsulated mass and was successful in stopping reflux[112]. Reflux ceased after one injection in 112 of 150 refluxing ureters, but, on follow up, it had recurred in 23 ureters, 8 of them with Grade II or IV reflux (IRSC grading). The procedure is simple and hospital admission time is shorter than for standard surgical techniques and clearly has great potential in the management of children with VUR. The long-term follow up will be of great interest. There are, however, some reservations about the use of Teflon in children in view of reports of migration of Teflon particles to other organs, including the lungs, meninges and lymph nodes, in canine experiments and also in man[113,114]. A chronic granulomatous reaction has been seen at the site of migration. Bovine collagen and other materials are being explored as an alternative to Teflon.

Controlled trials of medical and surgical management of children with VUR

The enthusiasm with which surgeons in the early 1960s embraced ureteric reimplantation together with YV plasty of the bladder neck, has been tempered by the recognition that some of the early operations carried both immediate and delayed complications from vesico-ureteric junction obstruction and that bladder neck obstruction was not usually the cause of reflux. The demonstration that all but the most severe vesico-ureteric reflux has a natural tendency to improve or disappear and the successful use of low-dose antibacterial prophylaxis in preventing recurrent UTI and allowing normal renal growth to occur, have also modified the management of these children. Where there was a good liaison between paediatric and surgical colleagues,

70

controlled studies of medical and surgical management of VUR were possible. Scott and Stansfeld[115] showed that successful surgery was marginally better than six months antibacterial treatment in preventing infection. White and Corkery set up the Birmingham Reflux Study; Williams, Ransley, Barratt and Dillon, at the Hospital for Sick Children, Great Ormond Street, concentrated on the infant with bilateral gross reflux. Olbing, with his surgical colleague, Professor Mellin, in Essen, successfully gathered groups of paediatric and surgical colleagues from Europe and America to collaborate in the International Reflux Study in Children[116]. Other trials are in progress.

Birmingham Study

In the Birmingham Study, children were eligible for entry who were aged less than 15 with reflux extending up to the kidney, either with calyceal distension or with renal scarring. Patients with duplex systems, horseshoe kidneys, severely impaired renal function or previous ureteric surgery were excluded[117]. Children were randomly allocated to operative or non-operative treatment and stratified for age into three groups. Continuous prophylaxis was prescribed in all. In the surgical group, two surgeons were involved and two techniques, Cohen and Leadbetter–Politano, were used. Postoperative follow up and also the management of the medical group were carried out by paediatric nephrologists and care was shared with peripheral referring paediatricians. The first follow up studies were made at two years. The results in 96 children showed no significant difference between the two groups in incidence of breakthrough infection, formation of new scars, progression of existing scars or in renal growth. There was a marginally significant improvement in overnight renal concentrating capacity of those surgically treated, but no differential renal function studies were included in the protocol.

The five-year follow-up appraisal of 104 of the children in the study (45%) has confirmed these findings[118]. Reflux was abolished in 98% of ureters reimplanted, but, although it persisted in more than half of those in children treated 'non-operatively', there was no significant difference in renal excretory function and concentrating ability between the two groups. Neither surgical nor non-operative man-

71

agement proved to be superior in the management of these children. Of particular interest, however, is the fact that, although there was some 'extension of existing scars', no new scars were detected between the two- and five-year follow up, whereas ten children developed new scars during the first two years. This would suggest that the scarring was initiated by the presenting infection before entry to the study, and, not only strongly supports Ransley and Risden's hypothesis that the main damage is inflicted during the first symptomatic infection, but emphasizes the importance of identifying those at risk before scarring develops.

Some of these children were included by kind permission of Dr White in our collaborative study of patients with fresh renal scarring[91]. A group of 18 kidneys from Birmingham showing new scars and 17 from UCH, all collected prospectively, underline that it is the *recognition and rapid treatment of the presenting infection in the child with the refluxing urinary tract which really matters* if the incidence of acquired reflux nephropathy is to be reduced. Since it has been shown that further new scars can develop in damaged kidneys, and over the age of 5 years, the prevention of symptomatic infection and the possibility of reflux-preventing surgery are still of major importance in these children throughout childhood.

The International Reflux Study in Children

The criteria for entry to the study were those with Grade III and IV reflux (International grading), aged 1–10 inclusive, without outflow obstruction or previous urinary tract surgery and without significant hypertension or renal failure. The groups were matched and stratified for age, sex and grade of reflux. Recruitment of over 400 children was completed in 1983 and the full results will not be analysed until the 5-year follow up has been completed[116]. The protocol of the European limb included a 3–6 months pre-allocation period on low-dose prophylaxis, after which the cystogram was repeated to confirm the grading. It is of some interest that, in 20% of the children randomized, reflux had either ceased or improved sufficiently for them to be ineligible for entry to the study. The second important finding was that when the rates for recurrent infection on prophylaxis in the pre-allocation period and postsurgery six months were compared with the same periods in the medical group, there was no significant difference in recurrence rate before and after surgery, or between medical and surgical groups. There was, however, significantly less febrile symptomatic infection after surgery[82].

A recent preliminary report of a controlled treatment trial of 90 children with VUR has confirmed that less severe grades of reflux can be managed satisfactorily with a medical regimen. The authors suggest that surgery should be considered for those with gross reflux[26].

THE NATURAL HISTORY OF VUR AND ITS SEQUELAE

The natural history of reflux in the human subject is unknown. A child investigated for urinary tract infection and found to reflux is usually treated. The natural course of events is thus immediately changed.

Figures for the causes of chronic renal failure (CRF), based on the European Dialysis and Transplant (EDTA) Programme and expressed as a percentage, depend on the accuracy of the diagnosis of reflux nephropathy and also reflect the accuracy of diagnosis and the proportions of other causes of CRF.

The lower percentage of CRF due to reflux nephropathy reported in Sweden, compared with other countries and the EDTA, may be due to the greater attention paid there to the recognition and rapid treatment of childhood UTI.

The Cardiff–Oxford Study of the treatment of schoolgirls with 'screening bacteriuria' included an untreated control group. Girls with VUR were included but not those with renal scarring. All girls were aged 5 years or over at the start. There was no difference in the persistence or recurrence of bacteriuria in untreated girls with or without reflux. When the differential renal function of a cohort of these girls was examined using the DTPA renogram, no significant difference in function was found in girls with or without reflux. The only factor significantly affecting renal function and therefore determining prognosis was the effective renal mass which was dependent on the presence or absence of renal scarring[119].

Reflux nephropathy and hypertension

Studies of severe hypertension in children have shown that one of the major causes is reflux nephropathy[120,121]. This association has long been recognized and the risk to children and young adults with renal scarring of developing hypertension has been assessed at 10–25%, the risk being greater when scarring is bilateral[67,68]. Renal hypertension seldom develops under the age of five years and other causes, such as coarctation of the aorta, must be considered in early childhood. Accelerated hypertension, however, is often due to reflux nephropathy, particularly if there are neurological complications.

The underlying mechanisms for developing renal hypertension have been explored in the last decade, particularly with regard to the renin–angiotensin system. Patients with reflux nephropathy and hypertension have been found to have raised plasma renin activity (PRA) in the renal veins draining a scarred kidney and in smaller segmental veins draining a scarred segment. The PRA has been less consistently raised in peripheral vein samples[122,123]. In a small series of 22 patients, nephrectomy or partial nephrectomy, removing a scarred area with raised plasma renin activity in the renal vein sample, was followed by a fall in blood pressure[123]. This provides an explanation for earlier observations that hypertension associated with unilateral renal scarring could be 'cured' by nephrectomy, which led for a time to 'prophylactic' nephrectomy. Similar benefits from surgery were noted by Stecker et al.[124] but these findings have not been confirmed by Bailey et al.[125].

Studies of the PRA in normotensive patients with reflux nephropathy suggested that a rise in PRA may antedate any rise in systemic blood pressure and thus could act as a marker for patients requiring careful follow up. However, Savage et al.[126], in a prospective follow-up study of a group of children with reflux nephropathy, did not find any consistent direct correlation between raised PRA levels and hypertension. They did show, however, during follow-up that the levels of circulating PRA in adolescence which tend to fall with age were sustained in the group of children with reflux nephropathy.

Lindeman et al.[127] and Bergström et al.[128] have shown in adult patients, not only that hypertension is closely associated with renal insufficiency, but also that a reduction in blood pressure has a beneficial effect on intraglomerular haemodynamics and delays glomerulo-sclerosis, whatever the aetiology, and progressive deterioration in renal function.

This provides support for the clinical impression that early therapy of even moderate levels of hypertension may prevent the onset, or delay the progress, of serious renal failure.

Clinical application: Patients with reflux nephropathy should have their blood pressure monitored regularly and annually at least, so that appropriate management can be instituted early.

Reflux nephropathy and reflux in adults

There have been few surveys of adults with reflux, but all point to the presence and severity of renal damage rather than the persistence of reflux as the main determinant of health and prognosis.

Hawtrey *et al.* reviewed 117 adolescent and adult patients with VUR, with ages ranging from 10–82 years and including patients with neuropathic bladders. They presented in a variety of ways and 49% had Grade III–V reflux (IRSC grading)[129]. From such a varied population, few conclusions can be drawn.

A number of studies of reflux nephropathy and its consequences in adults have been made[130–133]. In the patients investigated, about half have shown reflux: in the others it had either been corrected or was assumed to have stopped spontaneously. Both Gower[130] and the Portsmouth Group[131] found that symptomatic infection could be controlled by antibacterial treatment or prophylaxis, and, if this was done, the majority of patients remained clinically well. Arze *et al.* found no evidence that recurrent infection caused either a progressive decline in renal function or the development of new scars[132]. The characteristics which they found to be significantly related to slowly declining GFR were hypertension, bilateral renal disease and proteinuria. Three of 58 patients followed in Portsmouth and 22 of 130 in Newcastle showed deterioration, mostly under the age of 40[131,132]. Renal failure was present in 2 of 56 patients without VUR and 3 of 27 with reflux. This difference was not significant. Thus, in these reports, the patients with reflux nephropathy with or without reflux mainly followed a benign course.

Kincaid Smith's experience is less favourable. In 1975, she described glomerular lesions associated with reflux nephropathy in adults[134], and more recently with Becker, she has explored this and demonstrated a generalized focal and segmental glomerular hyalinosis and sclerosis which appears to become more widespread with age. This may not be apparent radiologically but is likely to contribute to the progression to renal failure seen in some patients[63,64,133]. Indicators of a poor prognosis which they identified included raised plasma creatinine, hypertension (which they found to be almost invariably present), moderate proteinuria (more than 1g day^{-1}) and grossly reduced renal substance on IVU. Factors which they found to accelerate deterioration include hypertension and pregnancy.

It is common clinical experience that once renal function has deteriorated to a certain point, further deterioration is inevitable, whether or not reflux is corrected, or infection is prevented or hypertension is controlled. A theory currently proposed for this is that there is hyperfiltration of the remaining functioning nephrons and this hyper-filtration results in progressive glomerular sclerosis and decline of renal function[135]. This may be amenable to therapy by reduction of dietary protein intake. For instance, in patients with a glomerular filtration rate (GFR) less than $40 \text{ ml min}^{-1} (1.73\text{m}^2)^{-1}$, minimizing the intake of dairy products will reduce protein and phosphate intake and appears to be beneficial.

The surgical correction of reflux plays little or no part in the management of adults unless there is uncontrollable symptomatic UTI[136].

CONCLUSION

Research over the past two decades has shown that vesico-ureteric reflux is usually congenital, often familial in incidence and, in most instances, self-limiting.

Clinically and experimentally, it has been shown to be closely linked with the pathogenesis of renal scarring by allowing a surge of pressure, with bacteria if the urine is infected, to reach the renal pelvis, calyces and papillae where an inflammatory response or pressure changes may damage the renal tissues, particularly if compound renal papillae are present. The consequence of this is renal scarring and impaired renal growth, with a risk of secondary hypertension or deteriorating renal function which may lead to end-stage renal failure. A small number will develop generalized focal and segmental glomerular changes accompanied by proteinuria and more rapid progression to end-stage renal disease.

Scarring develops almost exclusively in childhood, particularly in infants and younger children, but significant new scars can develop in normal and already scarred kidneys throughout childhood. Experienced surgeons can 'cure' reflux and careful medical supervision will prevent recurrent infection, but neither programme will affect the outcome if a first symptomatic infection is overlooked, inadequately treated or allowed to recur in susceptible individuals. Scarring is permanent and as cure is not possible, prevention is essential.

Specific research into aetiology has resulted in the screening of siblings and offspring of index reflux patients so they can be identified before damage has taken place. Research into diagnosis and investigation has led to the identification and follow up of infants with fetal dilatation of the urinary tract on antenatal ultrasound, to the recommendation of early diagnosis and rapid treatment of urinary tract infection in the febrile sick child and the use of tests, such as the C reactive protein or the DMSA scan, in children with symptomatic urinary tract infection to identify those likely to have renal involvement. Alternatives to contrast cystography, particularly for the follow up of children with VUR, have been developed. More parallel studies of these are required.

Research into the pathogenesis of renal scarring and the effect of the combination of urinary infection and reflux has pointed to the importance of rapid effective treatment of urinary tract infection, until it is known whether reflux is present, and vigilance in the prevention of further infection in those in whom reflux is demonstrated.

Although the results of controlled trials of the medical and surgical management of children with VUR have so far given no indication of the superiority of one method over the other, the management of each child should be planned individually and will depend upon circumstances, such as age, renal status and severity of reflux. Geo-

77

graphical location in relation to both appropriate medical care and supervision and experienced paediatric surgeons, the anticipated level of compliance by the child and the family and the result on follow up will all influence this.

Most surgical intervention in the future is likely to be carried out for either severe reflux or uncontrolled recurrent symptomatic infection, due to either medical or social reasons. Results are needed of further long-term studies of the outcome of both medical and surgical management, as well as of different surgical techniques.

Acknowledgements

Dr Smellie is very grateful for the support of The National Kidney Research Fund and for the secretarial help of Mrs Jan Port.

REFERENCES

1. Scott, J. E. S. (1975). The role of surgery in the management of vesico-ureteric reflux. *Kidney Int.,* **8,** S73–S80
2. Smellie, J. M. (1967). Medical aspects of urinary infection in children. *J. R. Coll. Physicians (London),* **1,** 189–196
3. Rolleston, G. L., Maling, T. M. J. and Hodson, C. J. (1974). Intrarenal reflux and the scarred kidney. *Arch. Dis. Child.,* **49,** 531–539
4. Shah, K. J. Robins, D. G. and White, R. H. (1978). Renal scarring and vesico-ureteric reflux. *Arch. Dis. Child.,* **53,** 210–217
5. Heikel, P. E. and Parkkulainen, K. V. (1966). Vesico-ureteric reflux in children: a classification and results of conservative treatment. *Ann. Radiol.,* **9,** 1–4
6. Dwoskin, J. Y. and Perlmutter, A. D. (1973). Vesico-ureteral reflux in children: a computerised review. *J. Urol.,* **109,** 888–890
7. International Reflux Study in Children (1985). International system of radiographic grading of vesico-ureteric reflux. *Pediatr. Radiol.,* **15,** 105–109
8. Sampson, J. A. (1903). Ascending renal infection with special reference to the reflux of urine from the bladder into the ureters as an aetiological factor in its causation and maintenance. *Bull. Johns Hopkins Hosp.,* **14,** 334–350
9. Bumpus, H. C. (1924). Urinary reflux. *J. Urol.,* **12,** 341–346
10. Iannacone, G. and Panzironi, P. E. (1965). Ureteral reflux in normal infants. *Acta Radiol.,* **44,** 451
11. Jones, P. W. and Headstream, J. W. (1958). Vesico-ureteral reflux in children. *J. Urol.,* **80,** 114–115
12. Lich, R, Howerton, L. W., Goode, L. S. and Davis, L. A. (1964). The ureterovesical junction of the newborn. *J. Urol.,* **92,** 436–438

13. Smellie, J. M., Hodson, C. J., Edwards, D. and Normand, I. C. S. (1964). Clinical and radiological features of urinary tract infection in childhood. *Br. Med. J.*, **2**, 1222–1226
14. Smellie, J. M., Normand, I. C. S. and Katz, G. (1981). Children with urinary infection: a comparison of those with and those without vesico-ureteric reflux. *Kidney Int.*, **20**, 717–722
15. McKerrow, W., Davidson-Lamb, N. and Jones, P. F. (1984). Urinary tract infection in children. *Br. Med. J.*, **289**, 299–303
16. Blickman, J. G., Taylor, G. A. and Lebowitz, (1985). Voiding cysto-urethrography: the initial radiological study in children with urinary tract infection. *Radiology*, **156**, 659–662
17. Kunin, C. M., Deutscher, R. and Paquin, A. (1964). Urinary tract infection in schoolchildren: an epidemiological clinical and laboratory study. *Medicine (Baltimore)*, **43**, 91–130
18. Verrier-Jones, K., Verrier-Jones, E. R. and Asscher, A. W. (1986). Covert urinary tract infections in children. In Asscher, A. W. and Brumfitt, W. (eds.) *Microbial Diseases in Nephrology*, Chapt. 14, pp. 225–239. (Chichester: John Wiley and Sons)
19. Askari, A. and Belman, A. B. (1982). VUR in black girls. *J. Urol.*, **127**, 747–748
20. Cremin, B. J. (1980). The many faces of primary vesico-ureteric reflux. *Pediatr. Radiol.*, **10**, 57
21. Baker, R., Maxted, W., Maylath, J. and Shuman, I. (1966). Relation of age, sex and infection to reflux: data indicating high spontaneous cure rate in paediatric patients. *J. Urol.*, **95**, 27–32
22. Smellie, J. M. (1969). The disappearance of reflux in children with urinary tract infection during prophylactic chemotherapy. *Proceedings of 4th International Congress of Nephrology*, Vol. 3, pp. 357–359, (Basel: S. Karger)
23. Reischauer, H-C., Olbing, H., Stroetges, M. W. and Kuehn, U. (1969). Disappearance of vesico renal reflux on conservative treatment. *German Med. Mon.*, **4**, 187–189
24. Stephens, F. D. (1972). Urologic aspects of recurrent urinary tract infection in children. *J. Pediatr.*, **80**, 725–737
25. King, L. R., Kazmi, S. O. and Belman, A. B. (1974). Natural history of vesico-ureteral reflux: outcome of a trial of non-operative therapy. *Urol. Clin. N. Am.*, **1**, 441–455
26. Scholtmeijer, R. J. and Griffiths, D. J. (1988). Treatment of vesico-ureteric reflux. Preliminary report of a prospective study. *Br. J. Urol.*, **61**, 205–209
27. Kleeman, C. R., Hewitt, W. L. and Guze, L. B. (1960). Pyelonephritis. *Medicine (Baltimore)*, **39**, 3–116
28. Hodson, C. J. and Edwards, D. (1960). Chronic pyelonephritis and vesico-ureteric reflux. *Clin. Rad.*, **11**, 219–231
29. Hutch, J. A., Miller, E. R. and Hinman, F. Jr. (1963). Vesico-ureteral reflux. Role in pyelonephritis. *Am. J. Med.*, **34**, 338–349
30. Normand, I. C. S. and Smellie, J. M. (1965). Prolonged maintenance chemotherapy in the management of urinary infection in childhood. *Br. Med. J.*, **1**, 1023–1026
31. Smellie, J. M. and Normand, I. C. S. (1968). Experience of follow-up of children with urinary tract infection. In O'Grady, F. and Brumfitt, W. (eds.) *Urinary Tract Infection*, pp. 123–138. (London: Oxford University Press)

32. Lyon, R. P., Marshall, S. and Tanagho, E. A. (1969). The ureteral orifice: its configuration and competence. *J. Urol.*, **102**, 504–509

33. Brock, W. A. and Kaplan, G. W. (1984). The value of endoscopy in deciding management of primary reflux. In Johnston, J. H. (ed.) *Management of Vesico-ureteric Reflux. International Perspectives in Urology*, Vol. 10. (Baltimore: Williams and Wilkins Co.)

34. Duckett, J. and Bellinger, M. F. (1984). Cystographic grading of primary reflux as an indicator of treatment. In Johnson, J. H. (ed.) *Management of Vesico-ureteric Reflux. International Perspectives in Urology*, Vol. 10. (Baltimore: Williams and Wilkins Co.)

35. Vermillion, C. D. and Heale, W. F. (1973). Position and configuration of the ureteral orifices and its relationship to renal scarring in adults. *J. Urol.*, **109**, 579–584

36. Stephens, F. D., Joske, R. A. and Simmons, R. T. (1955). Megaureter with vesico-ureteral reflux in twins. *Aust. N.Z. J. Surg.*, **24**, 192–4

37. Hayden, L. J. and Koff, S. A. (1984). Vesico ureteric reflux in triplets. *J. Urol.*, **132**, 516–517

38. Annotation (1975). Vesico ureteral reflux and its familial distribution. *Br. Med. J.*, **2**, 726

39. De Vargas, A., Evans, K., Ransley, P., Rosenberg, A. R., Rothwell, D., Sherwood, T., Williams, D. I., Barratt, T. M. and Carter, C. O. (1978). A family study of vesico-ureteric reflux. *J. Med. Genet.*, **15**, 85–96

40. Bailey, R. R., Janus, E., McLoughlin, K., Lynn, K. L. and Abbott, G. D. (1984). Familial and genetic data in reflux nephropathy. *Contr. Nephrol.*, **39**, 40–51

41. Atwell, J. D., Cook, P. L., Strong, L. and Hyde, I. (1977). The interrelationship between vesico-ureteric reflux, trigonal abnormalities and a bifid pelvicalyceal collecting system in a family study. *Br. J. Urol.*, **49**, 97–107

42. Goldraich, N. P., Goldraich, I. H., Anselmi, O. E. and Ramos, O. L. (1984). Reflux nephropathy: the clinical picture in South Brazilian children. *Contr. Nephrol.*, **39**, 52–67

43. Jerkins, G. R. and Noe, N. (1982). Familial vesico-ureteral reflux: a prospective study. *J. Urol.*, **128**, 774–777

44. Chapman, C. J., Bailey, R. R., Janus, E. D., Abbott, G. D. and Lynn, K. L. (1985). Vesico-ureteric reflux, segregation analysis. *Am. J. Med. Genet.*, **20**, 577–584

45. Allen, T. D. (1979). Vesico-ureteric reflux as a manifestation of dysfunctional voiding. In Hodson, J., and Kincaid Smith, P. (eds.) *Reflux Nephropathy*, pp. 171–180. (New York: Massson)

46. Van Gool, J. D., Kuitjen, R. H., Donckerwolcke, R. A., Messer, A. P. and Vijverberg, M. (1984). Bladder-sphincter dysfunction, urinary infection and vesico-ureteral reflux with special reference to cognitive bladder training. *Contr. Nephrol.*, **39**, 190–210

47. Woods, C. and Atwell, J. D. (1982). Vesico-ureteric reflux in the neuropathic bladder with particular reference to the development of renal scarring. *Eur. Urol.*, **8**, 23–28

48. Bauer, S. B., Retik, A. B., Colodny, A. H., Hallett, M., Khoshbin, S. and Dyro, F. M. (1980). The unstable bladder of childhood. *Urol. Clin. N. Am.*, **7**, 321–335

49. Taylor, C. M., Corkery, J. J. and White, R. H. R. (1982). Micturition symptoms

and unstable bladder activity in girls with primary vesico-ureteric reflux. *Br. J. Urol.*, **54**, 494–498

50. Alon, U., Pery, M., Davidai, G. and Berant, M. (1986). Ultrasonography in the evaluation of children with urinary tract infection. *Pediatrics*, **78**, 58–64

51. Thomas, D. F. M. (1984). Urological diagnosis in utero. *Arch. Dis. Child.*, **59**, 913–915

52. Grupe, W. (1987). The dilemma of intra-uterine diagnosis of congenital renal disease. *Ped. Clin. N. Am.*, **34**, 629–638

53. Smith, D., Egginton, J. A. and Brookfield, D. S. K. (1987). Detection of abnormality of fetal urinary tract as a predictor of renal tract disease. *Br. Med. J.*, **294**, 27–28

54. Lebowitz, R. L. (1986). The detection of vesico-ureteral reflux in the child. *Invest. Urol.*, **21**, 519–531

55. Majd, M. and Belman, A. B. (1979). Nuclear cystography in infants and children. *Urol. Clin. N. Am.*, **21**, 519–531

56. Conway, J. J. (1984). Radionuclide cystography. *Contr. Nephrol.*, **39**, 1–19

57. Chapman, S. J., Chantler, C., Haycock, G. B., Maisey, M. N. and Saxton, H. M. (1988). Is your cystogram really necessary? The role of indirect cystography in the detection and management of VUR. *Arch. Dis. Child.*, **63**, 650–651

58. Van den Abeele, A. D., Treves, S. T., Lebowitz, R. L., Bauer, S., Davis, R. T., Retik, A. and Colodny, A. (1987). Vesico-ureteral reflux in asymptomatic siblings of patients with known reflux: radionuclide cystography. *Pediatrics*, **79**, 147–153

59. Claësson, K., Jacobsson, B., Olsson, T. and Ringertz, H. (1981). Assessment of renal parenchymal thickness in normal children. *Acta Radiol. (Stockholm)*, **22**, 305–314

60. Merrick, V. M., Uttley, W. S. and Wild, S. R. (1980). The detection of pyelonephritis scarring in children by radio-isotope imaging. *Br. J. Radiol.*, **53**, 544–556

61. Sty, J. R., Wells, R. G., Starshak, R. J. and Schroeder, B. A. (1987). Imaging in acute renal infection in children. *Am. J. Roentgenol.*, **148**, 471–477

62. Smellie, J. M., Shaw, P. J., Prescod, N. P. and Bantock, H. M. (1988). ^{99m}Tc dimercapto-succinic acid scan in patients with established radiological renal scarring. *Arch. Dis. Child.*, **63**, 1315–1319

63. Kincaid Smith, P. (1984). Diffuse parenchymal lesions in reflux nephropathy and the possibility of making a renal biopsy diagnosis in reflux nephropathy. *Contr. Nephrol.*, **39**, 111–115

64. Kincaid Smith, P. and Becker, G. (1979). Reflux nephropathy in the adult. In Hodson, J. and Kincaid Smith, P. (eds) *Reflux Nephropathy*, pp. 21–28. (New York: Masson)

65. Smellie, J. M., Preece, M. A. and Paton, A. M. (1983). Normal somatic growth in children receiving low dose prophylactic co-trimoxazole. *Eur. J. Pediatr.*, **140**, 301–304

66. Donckerwolke, R. A. and Brunner, F. (1982). Combined report on regular dialysis and transplantation of children in Europe 1981. *Proc. Eur. Dial. Transplant. Assoc.*, **20**, 60–91

67. Wallace, D. M. A., Rothwell, D. L. and Williams, D. I. (1978). The long term follow up of surgically treated vesico-ureteric reflux. *Br. J. Urol.*, **50**, 479–484

68. Smellie, J. M. and Normand, I. C. S. (1979). Reflux nephropathy in childhood.

81

In Hodson, C. J. and Kincaid Smith, P. (eds) *Reflux Nephropathy*, pp. 14–20. (New York: Masson Publishing USA Inc.)

69. Hodson, J. and Kincaid Smith, P. (1979). *Reflux Nephropathy*, (New York: Masson Publishing USA Inc.)
70. Hodson, C. J., Heptinstall, R. H. and Winberg, J. (1984). *Reflux Nephropathy Update: 1983.* (Basel: S. Karger)
71. Hutch, J. A. and Smith, D. (1969). Sterile reflux: report of 24 cases. *Urol. Int.,* **24,** 460–665
72. Scott, D. J., Blackford, H. N., Joyce, M. R. L., Mundy, A. R., Kinder, C. H., Haycock, G. B. and Chantler, C. (1986). Renal function following surgical correction of vesico-ureteric reflux in childhood. *Br. J. Urol.,* **58,** 119–124
73. Aperia, A., Broberger, O., Ericsson, N. O. and Wikstad, I. (1976). Effect of vesico-ureteral reflux on renal function in children with recurrent infections. *Kidney Int.,* **9,** 418–423
74. Wikstad, I., Aperia, A., Broberger, O. and Ekengren, K. (1979). Vesico-ureteric reflux and pyelonephritis: long time effect on area of renal parenchyma. *Acta Radiol. Diag.,* **20,** 252–260
75. Mundy, A. R., Borzyskowski, M. and Saxton, H. M. (1982). Video urodynamic evaluation of neuropathic vesico-urethral dysfunction in children. *Br. J. Urol.,* **54,** 645–649
76. Smellie, J. M. and Normand, I. C. S. (1981). The natural history of reflux. In Gruskin, A. B. and Norman, M. E. (eds) *Pediatric Nephrology,* pp. 149–153. (The Hague: Martinus Nijhoff)
77. Hodson, C. J., Maling, T. M. J., McManamon, P. J. and Lewis, M. G. (1975). The pathogenesis of reflux nephropathy (Chronic Atrophic Pyelonephritis). *Br. J. Radiol. Suppl.,* **13,** 1–26
78. Ransley, P. G. and Risdon, R. A. (1978). Reflux and renal scarring. *Br. J. Radiol. Suppl.,* **14,** 1–34
79. Ransley, P. G., Risdon, R. A. and Godley, M. L. (1984). High pressure sterile vesicoureteral reflux and renal scarring: an experimental study in the pig and minipig. *Contr. Nephrol.,* **39,** 32–343
80. Ransley, P. G., Risdon, R. A. and Godley, M. L. (1987). Effects of vesico-ureteric reflux on renal growth and function as measured by GFR, plasma creatinine and urinary concentrating ability. *Br. J. Urol.,* **60,** 193–204
81. O'Grady, F. W. and Cattell, W. R. (1960). Kinetics of urinary tract infection. II. The Bladder. *Br. J. Urol.,* **38,** 156–158
82. Olbing, H. (1987). Vesico-uretero-renal reflux and the kidney. *Pediatr. Nephrol.,* **1,** 638–646
83. Elo, J., Tallgren, L. G., Alfthan, O. and Sarna, S. (1983). Character of urinary tract infections and pyelonephritic renal scarring after antireflux surgery. *J. Urol.,* **129,** 343–346
84. Smellie, J. M. and Prescod, N. (1986). Overt urinary tract infection in childhood. In Asscher, A. W. and Brumfitt, W. (eds) *Microbial Diseases in Nephrology.* (Chichester: J. Wiley & Sons Ltd)
85. Smellie, J. M., Edwards, D., Hunter, N., Normand, I. C. S. and Prescod, N. (1975). Vesico-ureteric reflux and renal scarring. *Kidney Int.,* **8,** S65–S72
86. Ransley, P. G. and Risdon, R. A. (1981). Reflux nephropathy: effects of anti-microbial therapy on the evolution of the early pyelonephritic scar. *Kidney Int.,* **20,** 733–742

87. Smellie, J. M. and Normand, I. C. S. (1985). Urinary tract infection 1985. *Postgrad. Med. J.*, **61**, 895–905
88. Miller, T. and Phillips, S. (1981). Pyelonephritis: the relationship between infection, renal scarring and antimicrobial therapy. *Kidney Int.*, **19**, 654–662
89. Winberg, J., Bollgren, L., Källenius, G., Möllby, R. and Svenson, S. B. (1982). Clinical pyelonephritis and focal renal scarring. *Pediatr. Clin. N. Am.*, **29**, 801–813
90. Winter, A. L., Hardy, B. E., Alton, D. J., Arbus, G. S. and Churchill, B. M. Acquired renal scars in children. *J. Urol.*, **129**, 1190–1194
91. Smellie, J. M., Ransley, P. G., Normand, I. C. S., Prescod, N. and Edwards, D. (1985). Development of new renal scars: a collaborative study. *Br. Med. J.*, **290**, 1957–1960
92. Lenaghan, D., Whitaker, J. G., Jensen, F. and Stevens, F. D. (1976). The natural history of reflux and long-term effects of reflux on the kidney. *J. Urol.*, **115**, 728–730
93. Ransley, P. G. and Risdon, R. A. (1975). Renal papillary morphology in infants and young children. *Urol. Res.*, **3**, 111–113
94. Tamminen, T. E. and Kaprio, E. A. (1977). The relation of the shape of renal papillae and of collecting duct openings to intrarenal reflux. *Br. J. Urol.*, **49**, 345–353
95. Cremin, B. J. (1979). Observations on vesicoureteric reflux and intrarenal reflux: a review and survey of material. *Clin. Radiol.*, **30**, 607–621
96. Bellinger, M. F. (1965). The management of vesico-ureteric reflux. *Urol. Clin. N. Am.*, **12**, 23–29
97. Edwards, D., Normand, I. C. S., Prescod, N. and Smellie, J. M. (1977). Disappearance of vesico-ureteric reflux during long term prophylaxis of urinary tract infection in children. *Br. Med. J.*, **2**, 285–288
98. Smellie, J. M., Edwards, D., Normand, I. C. S. and Prescod, N. (1981). Effect of vesico-ureteric reflux on renal growth in children with urinary tract infection. *Arch. Dis. Child.*, **56**, 593–600
99. Skoog, S. J., Belman, A. B. and Majd, M. (1987). A non-surgical approach to the management of primary vesico-ureteral reflux. *J. Urol.*, **138**, 941–946
100. Smellie, J. M., Grüneberg, R. N., Leakey, A. and Atkin, W. S. (1976). Long-term low-dose co-trimoxazole in prophylaxis of childhood urinary tract infection: clinical aspects. *Br. Med. J.*, **2**, 203–206
101. Smellie, J. M., Grüneberg, R. N., Bantock, H. and Prescod, N. (1988). Prophylactic co-trimoxazole and trimethoprim in the management of urinary tract infection in children. *Pediatr. Nephrol.*, **2**, 12–17
102. Aladjem, M., Boichis, H., Hertz, M., Herzfeld, S. and Raviv, U. (1980). The conservative management of vesico-ureteral reflux: a review of 121 children. *Pediatrics*, **65**, 78–80
103. Homsey, Y. L., Nsouli, I., Hamburger, B., Laberge, I. and Schick, E. (1985). Effects of oxybutynin on vesico-ureteral reflux in children. *J. Urol.*, **134**, 1168–1171
104. Koff, S. A. and Murtagh, D. S. (1987). The uninhibited bladder in children. Effect of treatment on recurrence of urinary infection and on vesico ureteric reflux resolution. *J. Urol.*, **130**, 1139–1141
105. Allen, T. D. (1985). Vesico-ureteral reflux and the unstable bladder. *J. Urol.*, **134**, 1180

106. Bellinger, M. F. and Duckett, J. W. (1984). Vesico-ureteral reflux: a comparison of non-surgical and surgical management. *Contr. Nephrol.*, **39**, 81–93

107. Carpentier, P. J., Bettink, P. J., Hop, W. C. J. and Schroder, F. H. (1982). Reflux: a retrospective study of 100 ureteric reimplantations by the Politano–Leadbetter method and 100 by the Cohen technique. *Br. J. Urol.*, **54**, 230–233

108. Coleman, J. W. and McGovern, J. H. (1979). A 20 year experience of pediatric ureteral reimplantation: surgical results in 701 children. In Hodson, J. and Kincaid Smith, P. (eds) *Reflux Nephropathy*, pp. 299–305. (New York: Masson)

109. Teague, N. and Boyarsky, S. (1968). Further effects of coliform organisms on ureteral peristasis. *J. Urol.*, **99**, 720–724

110. Roberts, J. A. (1975). Experimental pyelonephritis in the monkey. III. Pathophysiology or ureteral malfunction induced by bacteria. *Invest. Urol.*, **13**, 117–120

111. Jörgenson, T. M. (1985). Dynamics of the urinary tract in long-term vesicoureteral reflux in pigs III. *Scand. J. Urol. Nephrol.*, **19**, 183–191

112. O'Donnell, B. and Puri, P. (1986). Endoscopic correction of primary vesicoureteric reflux. *Br. J. Urol.*, **58**, 601–604

113. Malizia, A. A., Reiman, H. M., Myers, R. P., Sande, J. R., Barham, S. S., Benson, R. C., Dewanjee, M. K. and Utz, W. J. (1984). Migration and granulomatous reaction after periurethral injection of politef (Teflon). *J. Am. Med. Assoc.*, **251**, 3277–3281

114. Mittleman, R. E. and Marraccini, J. V. (1983). Pulmonary Teflon granulomas following periurethral Teflon injection for urinary incontinence. *Arch. Pathol. Lab. Med.*, **107**, 611–612

115. Scott, J. E. S. and Stansfeld, J. M. (1968). Treatment of vesico-ureteric reflux in children. *Arch. Dis. Child.*, **43**, 323–328

116. International Reflux Study Committee (1980). Medical versus surgical treatment of primary vesico-ureteral reflux. *Pediatrics*, **67**, 392–400

117. Birmingham Reflux Study Group (1983). Prospective trial of operative versus non-operative treatment of severe vesico-ureteric reflux: two years' observation in 96 children. *Br. Med. J.*, **287**, 171–174

118. Birmingham Reflux Study Group (1987). A prospective trial of operative versus non-operative treatment of severe vesico-ureteric reflux: 5 years observation. *Br. Med. J.*, **295**, 237–241

119. Verrier-Jones, K., Asscher, A. W., Verrier-Jones, E. R., Mattholie, K, Leach, K. and Thomson, G. M. (1982). Glomerular filtration rate in schoolgirls with covert bacteriuria. *Br. Med. J.*, **285**, 1307–1310

120. Still, L. J. and Cottom, D. (1967). Severe hypertension in childhood. *Arch. Dis. Child.*, **42**, 34–39

121. Gill, D. G., Mendes da Costa, B., Cameron, J. S., Joseph, M. C., Ogg, C. S. and Chantler, C. (1976). Analysis of 100 children with severe and persistent hypertension. *Arch. Dis. Child.*, **51**, 951–956

122. Savage, J. M., Dillon, M. J., Shah, V., Barratt, T. M. and Williams, D. I. (1978). Renin and blood pressure in children with renal scarring and vesicoureteric reflux. *Lancet*, **2**, 441–444

123. Dillon, M. J. and Smellie, J. M. (1984). Peripheral plasma renin activity, hypertension and renal scarring in children. *Contr. Nephrol.*, **39**, 68–80

124. Stecker, J. F., Read, B. P. and Poutasse, E. F. (1977). Pediatric hypertension as

a delayed sequela of reflux-induced chronic pyelonephritis. *J. Urol.*, **118,** 644–646

125. Bailey, R. R., McRae, C. U., Maling, T. M.J., Tisch, G. and Little, P. J. (1978). Renal vein renin concentration in the hypertension of unilateral reflux nephropathy. *J. Urol.*, **120,** 21–23

126. Savage, J. M., Koh, C. T., Shah, V., Barratt, T. M. and Dillon, M. J. (1987). Five year prospective study of plasma renin activity and blood pressure in patients with longstanding reflux nephropathy. *Arch. Dis. Child.*, **62,** 678–682

127. Lindeman, R. D., Tobin, J. D. and Shock, N. W. (1984). Association between blood pressure and the rate of decline in renal function with age. *Kidney Int.*, **26,** 861–868

128. Bergström, J., Alvestrand, A., Bucht, H. and Gutierrez, A. (1988). Hypertension and its control in progressive renal failure. In Davidson, A. M. (ed.) *Nephrology*, Vol. II, pp. 1192–1196. (London: Bailliere Tindall)

129. Hawtrey, C. E., Culp, D. A., Loening, S., Fallon, B. and Maynard, M. (1983). Ureterovesical reflux in an adolescent and adult population. *J. Urol.*, **130,** 1067–1069

130. Gower, P. E. (1976). A prospective study of patients with radiological pyelonephritis, papillary necrosis and obstructive atrophy. *Q. J. Med.*, **178,** 315–349

131. Mihindukulasuriya, J. C. L., Maskell, R. and Polak, A. (1980). A study of fifty-eight patients with renal scarring associated with urinary tract infection. *Q. J. Med.*, **49,** 165–178

132. Arze, R. S., Ramos, J. M., Owen, J. P., Morley, A. R., Elliott, R. W., Wilkinson, R., Ward, M. K. and Kerr, D. N. S. (1982). The natural history of chronic pyelonephritis in the adult. *Q. J. Med.*, **204,** 396–410

133. Kincaid Smith, P. and Becker, G. (1978). Reflux nephropathy and chronic atrophic pyelonephritis. *J. Infect. Dis.*, **138,** 774–780

134. Kincaid Smith, P. (1975). Glomerular lesions in atrophic pyelonephritis and reflux nephropathy. *Kidney Int.*, **8** (Suppl. 4), S81–S83

135. Brenner, B. M., Meyer, T. W. and Hostetter, T. H. (1982). Dietary protein intake and the progressive nature of kidney disease: the role of haemodynamically mediated glomerular injury in the pathogenesis of progressive glomerular sclerosis in ageing, renal ablation and intrinsic renal disease. *N. Engl. J. Med.*, **307,** 652–659

136. Nativ, O., Hertz, M., Hanani, Y., Many, M. and Jonas, P. (1987). Vesico ureteral reflux in adults: a review of 95 patients. *Eur. Urol.*, **13,** 229–232

3

URINARY TRACT INFECTION IN OLD AGE

D. J. PROPPER

INTRODUCTION

Urinary tract infection (UTI) is one of the commonest disorders affecting the elderly population. Surprisingly, the problem has not been the subject of extensive investigation and its significance remains an enigma. Recently, however, there have been a number of reports from which have arisen contrasting views on its significance, especially with respect to mortality, morbidity, and the indications and efficacy of antimicrobial therapy. Perhaps this is not surprising as the elderly are a heterogeneous population; hence, the results of epidemiological surveys and therapeutic trials will vary according to which groups arc scrutinized, and, therefore, should be interpreted with caution. Furthermore, the elderly are already subject to considerable morbidity and mortality, so that any sequelae of UTI may be difficult to detect.

It is important to remember that significant bacteriuria is a statistical concept, introduced by Kass in order to distinguish contaminated urine from UTI[1], and originally applied to symptomless females with an isolate of 10^5 or more common urinary pathogens. This criterion may not be applicable when other organisms are cultured or in different population samples. This is especially relevant in the elderly, as the incidence of less common aerobic organisms, anaerobes and true mixed infections is greater than at younger ages [2-5]. Investigations of the elderly have almost exclusively depended on this criterion for diagnosing UTI. Many of the reports from which views on the nature of UTI in old age are based may, therefore, have erroneously categorized patients as abacteriuric.

Furthermore, in one study, patients' urine was cultured before and after a provoked diuresis and 50% of those with initially sterile urine had significant cultures during diuresis[6]. Conversely, in certain reports, patients have been classified as bacteriuric using inadequate diagnostic criteria, such as on the basis of a single urine culture. These caveats have to be borne in mind when interpreting the literature.

PREVALENCE

In old age, UTI is more widespread than at any other time of life and the marked sex difference of earlier years is less apparent. Amongst schoolgirls, the prevalence is between 1 and 2%, and steadily rises by approximately 1% each decade, until around 60, thereafter becoming increasingly common[7]. By the age of 70 years, the prevalence of UTI is around 20% for females[8,9]. In males, UTI is rare until the eighth decade, affecting only 3% of males between 65 and 70 years old[10], compared with 20% of those over the age of 80[9]. These prevalence rates are derived from population-based surveys. The prevalence, however, varies with the health of the group studied, and correlates with increasing degrees of infirmity and institutionalization[11]; approximately a quarter to one-third of male and female residents of old peoples' homes[11,12], and elderly hospital admissions[13] have UTI.

In long-stay institutions, infection rates are highest of all, with up to half the patients having UTI[3,14,15]. Moreover, the sex difference apparent amongst the elderly living independently weakens with the degree of infirmity and institutionalization, such that rates in institutions are similar for both sexes. (See Table 3.1.)

A much larger section of the geriatric population is affected by UTI than the figures in Table 3.1 at first suggest. This is because the number of elderly patients affected by UTI steadily rises with time, but the prevalence remains fairly static[11,16,17]. For instance, in the survey of elderly ambulatory patients by Boscia et al., the number of patients with UTIs, over an eighteen-month period, was almost double the prevalence[11]. The overall prevalence of UTI during that time, however, was unchanged. In most instances, the UTIs resolved spontaneously.

TABLE 3.1   Review of the prevalence of UTI in the elderly*

Group studied	Age (Years)	Prevalance (%)	
		Females	Males
Population survey			
Akhtar[46]	65+	17	6
Brocklehurst et al.[9]	65+	20	13
Heinamaki et al.[28]	85+	30	13
Nordenstam et al.[5]	70	9	2.4
Sourander[8]	65+	33	11
Residents of Old Persons Homes			
Boscia et al.[11]	68+	23% overall	
Dontas et al.[12]	70+	27	14
Hospital admissions			
Gibson and Pritchard[15]	60+	34	30
Walkey et al.[13]	60+	34	31
Wolfson et al.[4]	63 (median)	—	15
Residents in long-term care			
Bentzen and Vejlsgaard[25]	78 (mean)	31	15
Brocklehurst et al.[24]	—		
		34% overall	
Nicolle et al.[3]	80 (median)	—	33%

* Does not include patients with catheters

Furthermore, patients were only assessed at six-monthly intervals, which almost certainly led to an underestimation of the incidence. From this study and others, it appears that there are two populations of elderly patients with UTI. A small group, with persistent infection, and a much larger one, with intermittent infection. In this latter group, UTIs generally resolve spontaneously, and, if recurrence occurs, it is often with a different organism[18,19].

PATHOGENESIS

In the elderly, many factors which predispose to UTI at all ages are common – urinary tract instrumentation, urinary tract obstruction, calculus disease, and genito-urinary surgery. These factors do not, however, fully explain the ubiquitous nature of UTI in old age, and many patients have no obvious predisposition. Indeed, such factors would appear to be less important in the elderly than in other age groups[4]. Compared with younger adults, renal blood flow is reduced by 50% and glomerular filtration rate by 30%[20], and immune responses are less efficient[21]. Such changes perhaps impair resistance to renal colonization. These abnormalities do not, however, emerge as major aetiological processes for UTI[21], and it seems likely that UTI has a multifactorial pathogenesis in old age. Also, because the incidence of UTI varies between the sexes, so too must the aetiology. In males, anatomical and physiological changes in the prostate[22,23], and in females ageing pelvic musculature and connective tissue, as well as atrophy of the vaginal and periurethral epithelium have been implicated[7]. As at younger ages, haematogenous sources are rare and infection is almost exclusively due to ascending gut-derived bacteria. The following conditions are thought to contribute to the prevalence of UTI in the elderly.

Dementia

There is a strong association between declining intellect and UTI, and manifestations such as memory loss and impaired ability to perform daily living activities correlate with UTI[11]. Several studies have found that UTI is most common amongst patients with dementia, and infection rates of over 70% have been described in long-stay geriatric wards[3,24,25]. Just why impaired intellectual function is so often accompanied by UTI is unclear. When faecal or urinary incontinence complicate dementia, infection may be related to perineal colonization by bacteria, as Stamey and others have shown that, in women, such colonization often precedes UTI[26,27]. No relationship has been detected, however, between urinary incontinence and UTI in subjects with sufficient intellectual capacity to live independently[9], although

this has been found in long-stay hospital patients[24]. Perineal contamination, therefore, cannot be the entire explanation for the prevalence of UTI in patients with dementia.

Immobility

It has been suggested that immobility predisposes to UTI[16,28], possibly
because it leads to infrequent bladder voiding and urinary stasis, but
there is little evidence to support this concept. Studies which have
found a relationship have been population-based surveys, and have
probably compared patients in the community with patients in institutions, who are likely to be less mobile[16,28].

Institutionalized elderly patients are, however, more likely to have
some degree of intellectual impairment, which is associated with UTI.
Surveys comparing patients within institutions have either shown no
relationship or even a lower incidence of UTI in patients with impaired
mobility[24,25]. It is likely that this was because the more mobile patients
had features of dementia, whilst the less mobile ones had other physical
disabilities requiring institutional care[24].

Age-related changes in the urogenitalia

In the elderly female, urethral, vaginal and uterine prolapse are
common. Whether such prolapse predisposes to UTI is disputed.
Several studies have failed to demonstrate any relationship between
prolapse and UTI[24,29], whereas others[14,30] have, and a strong association has been reported between UTI and even slight vaginal laxity[14].
If such a relationship exists, the mechanism could be due to defective
sealing of the short female urethra, because no association has been
found between prolapse and urinary obstruction, or the presence of
residual postmicturation urine. It is not known whether prolapse
repair reduces the incidence of UTI in old age.

Although the presence of residual postmicturition urine, in the
absence of bladder neck obstruction, is widespread in the elderly, it
does not appear to correlate with infection[24]. Just why bladder
emptying is defective in old age is unclear, although Brocklehurst and

Dillane proposed that, with increasing age, there is a tendency to develop an uninhibited neurogenic bladder[31]. Whatever the cause, it is surprising that residual urine does not appear to result in infection, given that urine is a good culture medium. In the presence of bladder neck obstruction, for example, due to prostatic hypertrophy, infection readily develops.

After the menopause, atrophy of the vaginal and urethral epithelium parallel changes in pelvic musculature and connective tissue. Such atrophy may impair local immunity to bacterial colonization. Colonization of the perineum and introitus is thought to predispose to recurrent UTI in females[26,27]. Such colonization is said to be rare at low vaginal pH[32,33] and it has been suggested that oestrogen lowers vaginal pH by stimulating local acid production[32]. The prevalence of UTI rises sharply after the menopause and this phenomenon may be related to an increase in vaginal pH consequent on low post-menopausal oestrogen levels[34,35].

In addition, Reid *et al.* have proposed that the postmenopausal rise in incidence of UTI occurs partly because low oestrogen levels are associated with increased epithelial adherence to pathogenic *Escherichia coli*[36], although this has not been confirmed by others[37]. It has also been proposed that, in old age, levels of uromucoid (Tamm–Horsfall glycoprotein) secretion are reduced, possibly impairing resistance to bacterial colonization[38].

In males, age-related changes in the prostate contribute to many UTIs. The prostate enlarges throughout adult life, such that 75% of males over the age of 65 have evidence of bladder neck obstruction[39], which may cause urinary stasis and therefore UTI. In addition, with increasing age, the antibacterial properties of prostatic secretions are thought to decline[40]. Once infection is established in the prostate, it is difficult to treat, partly because most antibiotics penetrate the prostate poorly, and because many elderly men have prostatic microcalculi[40] which form an almost ineradicable source of bacteria. Furthermore, because of prostatic disease, elderly men are often subjected to urinary tract instrumentation and operations, which in turn predispose to UTI[9,25], suggesting that the prostate becomes colonized during such procedures. Interestingly, pelvic operations do not appear to predispose to infection in women[9].

Diabetes mellitus

With age, diabetes mellitus becomes increasingly common and the prevalence of UTI in adult women (but not men) with diabetes mellitus is said to be increased[41]. The proposed mechanisms include impaired bladder emptying consequent on diabetic neuropathy, impaired resistance to infection, and the favourable culture conditions of urine containing glucose. In both large community[5,28] and hospital surveys[42], however, the incidence of UTI was no greater amongst elderly diabetics.

Urinary catheters

Long-term bladder catheterization almost invariably causes UTI. Condom catheters are sometimes used in an attempt to circumvent this problem. Whilst this appears to be successful in the short term for co-operative patients[43], in the long term there is a high rate of infection[44]. With unco-operative patients, UTI rapidly supervenes, probably because of intermittent obstruction caused by manipulation of the collecting system. Furthermore, condom catheters may form reservoirs of bacteria and have been associated with outbreaks of infection[45].

SYMPTOMS

Apart from the occasional patient, UTI rarely presents in the elderly with the classical features of dysuria, loin pain, and frequency[8,9,25,46,47]. In fact, UTI is generally asymptomatic and a chance finding on urine culture. The elderly often have urinary symptoms, such as urgency, nocturia and frequency, whether or not they have infected urine[9] and, although such symptoms have been found with increased frequency amongst bacteriuric subjects, the increase is not marked[5]. In Brocklehurst et al.'s survey of elderly patients in the community, none of the urinary symptoms in males correlated with UTI and only for females with precipitancy and difficulty in passing urine was there any correlation with UTI[9]. Furthermore, although it has often been suggested that UTI presents in more subtle ways in the elderly – with such diverse symptoms as anorexia, fatigue, confusion, falls, malaise and insomnia – there is little evidence to support these views[48–50]. In fact, in a survey of patients in sheltered care, both urinary symptoms and symptoms of lack of well being were assessed during episodes of infection and when abacteriuric (either as a result of antimicrobial therapy or spontaneous resolution). No difference in symptoms was observed when patients had either sterile or infected urine[47]. The frequency of urinary symptoms in the elderly appears to be much more a consequence of age-related changes, such as prostatic hypertrophy and pelvic prolapse, than infection[9].

DIAGNOSIS

Diagnostic criteria

As in younger age groups, UTI is diagnosed on the criterion of 10^5 or more colony-forming units per ml of urine. As with all diagnostic tests, however, the application of a blanket criterion for positivity which was derived from a specific population has led to substantial confusion and erroneous diagnoses. Furthermore, in the general population, the isolation of 10^5 or more colony-forming units per ml of urine only indicates with 80% confidence that UTI is present[92].

Statistically, the diagnostic accuracy of MSSUs increases with the number collected. Two MSSUs are said to be 97% accurate and three almost 100% accurate[52]. Hence, before UTI is diagnosed in elderly patients, at least two positive MSSUs should be obtained and the same organism should be cultured on each occasion. One study has, however, suggested that as many as one-half of geriatric patients with conventionally obtained negative urine cultures may in fact have UTI[6]. In that study, of patients from a residential home, 47% of females with persistently sterile urine developed significant bacteriuria during a provoked diuresis. Fluorescent antibody-coating tests of the bacteria were positive in almost all instances, indicating that most of these patients harboured infection within the renal parenchyma. Conversely, many elderly patients receive diuretic medication, which may, by urinary dilution, lead to false negative cultures in cases of lower urinary tract infection.

A further source of confusion has been the loose application of terms such as 'cystitis' or 'bacteriuria'. In order to clarify this situation, the MRC Bacteriuria Committee has produced a recommended terminology (Table 3.2)[91].

Collection of urine

Collection of MSSUs from elderly females is often technically more demanding than from males, and is associated with higher rates of false positive results[25]. With co-operative patients, the vulva should be cleansed using sterile saline, and held apart whilst an MSSU is obtained by pressing a sterile beaker below the urethra. The collected urine is then poured out over a part of the rim that has not been in contact with the vulva. For less co-operative females the collection can be performed by two assistants with the patient sitting on a commode, or, for males, by using a condom catheter. If these manœuvres are unsuccessful and urine cultures are essential, the patient should be catheterized, although this in itself predisposes to infection. Bentzen and Vejlsgaard showed that, even in psychogeriatric wards, it is possible in almost all instances to obtain uncontaminated MSSUs if the collection is carried out by trained personnel[25]. Suprapubic collection, although rapid and safe, is, therefore, only rarely indicated. Moreover, it is uncomfortable and, in some hands, has only a 67% success rate[51].

Brocklehurst et al. correlated the diagnostic accuracy of MSSUs with specimens obtained by catheter and suprapubic puncture from females in long-stay geriatric wards and found that 17% of MSSUs were falsely positive[24], and Moore-Smith found that 57% of MSSUs from a similar group of patients were false positive[52]. This disparity probably reflects the care with which MSSUs were obtained.

In the elderly, pyuria is not sufficiently specific for diagnostic purposes. On urinary microscopy, Akhtar et al.[46] found that only 31% of elderly patients with significant bacteriuria had more than 3 white blood cells per high power field (HPF), whereas Brocklehurst et al.[9] found 79% had more than 4 white cells per HPF, and Sourander[8] found 63% had more than 10 white cells per mm[3]. The reasons for these discrepancies are not clear. However, sterile pyuria is common

TABLE 3.2   Clinical and bacteriological definition of urinary tract infections

Urinary tract infections	The presence of micro-organisms in the urinary tract.
Bacteriuria	The presence of bacteria in bladder urine.
Covert bacteriuria	Significant bacteriuria detected by the screening of apparently healthy populations. This term is preferred to symptomatic bacteriuria.
Upper-tract bacteriuria	The presence of bacteria in urine collected from the renal pelvis or ureter. This may indicate renal infection but, in the presence of vesicoureteric reflux, the organisms may derive from the bladder.
Frequency/dysuria syndrome	A clinical syndrome often called cystitis consisting of frequency and dysuria. Bladder bacteriuria may or may not be present.
Bacterial cystitis	A syndrome consisting of dysuria and frequency of micturition by day and night. Bladder bacteriuria is present and usually associated with pyuria and sometimes haematuria.
Abacterial cystitis	A syndrome consisting of dysuria and frequency in the absence of bladder bacteriuria. The use of the term urethral syndrome for this condition is not recommended as there is no evidence of urethral disease in most patients.
Acute bacterial pyelonephritis	A syndrome consisting of loin pain, tenderness and pyrexia accompanied by bacteriuria, bacteraemia, pyuria and sometimes haematuria. It is associated with bacterial infection of the kidney.

in the elderly. In a survey of 561 elderly subjects in the community, 50% had pyuria but only 25% had bacteriuria[28]. As pyuria can result from analgesic nephropathy, steroid therapy, tuberculosis, chronic prostatitis, chronic pyelonephritis, and other structural abnormalities of the renal parenchyma, all of which are found with increased frequency in the elderly, this high incidence is perhaps not surprising[53].

Further investigations

Adjunctive laboratory tests, such as creatinine, haemoglobin, leucocyte count and ESR, are generally normal[8,28,46]. Given the extensive prevalence of UTI, radiological investigation of the urological tract cannot be advocated for all patients with UTI as relatively few treatable lesions will be detected. Patients with persistent infection, symptoms of calculus or prostatic disease, and those who develop pyelonephritis should undergo ultrasound or radiological investigation as these are often associated with correctable structural abnormalities[54].

SITE OF INFECTION

The site of infection in the urinary tract has not been well defined in the elderly and it has often been assumed, without good evidence, that infection is usually confined to the lower urinary tract[14,46]. The findings of Suntharalingham et al. suggest that such assumptions may be incorrect[55]. Using a modification of the Fairley bladder washout technique to localize the site of infection[56], over one-half of female admissions to a geriatric unit had evidence of renal infection. The site of infection has not been defined in an unselected population of elderly males, but Smith et al.'s study of army veterans with recurrent UTI, many of whom were over 65 (mean age 69 years old), indicated that all had evidence of tissue involvement, with about half localizing to the prostate and half to the kidneys[57].

BACTERIA

In old age, UTIs are usually due to gut derived Gram-negative entero-bacteria. Infection with enterococci is, however, more prevalent than at younger ages[3,5,58]. Although *E. coli* is the most frequently isolated organism, it is less prevalent than at younger ages. *E. coli* accounts for 70–80% of UTIs affecting elderly subjects living at home, with other Gram-negative enterobacteria, particularly *Proteus miribilis,* accounting for most of the remainder[46]. With increasing disability, and in hospital, the microbial spectrum alters radically, and *Proteus mirabilis, Pseudomonas aeruginosa* and *Klebsiella* spp. are isolated much more frequently[2,3,13,46]. In Akhtar *et al.*'s series[46], *E. coli* accounted for 71% of out-patient UTIs and *P. miribilis* for 7%, whereas, in hospital, *E. coli* caused only 50% and *P. miribilis* 39%[46]. Furthermore, amongst elderly in-patients, mixed urinary cultures are common [2–5] – 39% of Nicolle's non-catherized male patients in long-term care had mixed cultures on repeated testing[3]. A tendency to discount mixed culture results as contamination should therefore be resisted.

It is not fully understood why the microbial spectrum alters with age, but structural changes in the renal tract, such as pyelonephritis and carcinoma, are associated with mixed urine cultures, and calculus disease may be associated with *proteus miribilis* infection[58]. The altered spectrum in hospital may also reflect excessively liberal antibiotic policies for treating UTI.

THE RELATIONSHIP OF UTI TO EXCESS MORTALITY

One of the crucial aspects concerning UTI in the elderly is whether it is associated with excess mortality. Even supposing that such a relationship exists, then is UTI a direct cause of excess mortality or is it simply associated with diseases which are? Furthermore, even if it were convincingly shown that UTI adversely affects life expectancy, is there evidence that treatment can reverse this effect? The literature is controversial on these aspects and must, therefore, be examined in some detail.

There have been four surveys assessing the contribution of UTI to mortality rates in the elderly[5,12,16,18]. The survey reported by Nicolle *et al.* dealt with males in long-stay geriatric wards and showed that mortality was no greater amongst patients with UTI than for non-infected patients[18]. The survey by Sourander and Kasanen, of a representative sample of the population, found that mortality rates were increased only amongst women between the ages of 75 and 79 years[16]. Only in the study by Dontas *et al.*, on ambient patients in a nursing home, was mortality reported to be greater for patients of both sexes with UTI[12]. Admittedly, Nordenstam *et al.*'s survey of a representative sample of the population over the age of 70 years found increased mortality rates in males with UTI, and a trend, which was not statistically significant, towards excess mortality for women with UTI[5]. When the data for catheterized females and for males with genito-urinary malignancy were discounted, however, life expectancy was not decreased for patients with UTI.

The results of these studies are, therefore, conflicting and inconclusive, and have been the subject of several major criticisms. The Dontas study has been criticized because, amongst the bacteriuric group, there was an excess of deaths due to cerebrovascular disease and 'senile cachexia', both of which could have been associated with dementia. It is known that dementia is associated with UTI[24] and also with excess mortality[59]. Moreover, as was pointed out by Kirkland and Robinson, the patients over 80 years old in Dontas *et al.*'s bacteriuric group had similar mortality rates to those predicted in patients of a similar age with dementia[60]. The observed excess mortality rates in the patients with UTI could therefore have been because they were more affected by dementia.

Nordenstam *et al.* have criticized the studies of Dontas *et al.* and Sourander and Kasanen because their subjects were grouped into age strata with a range of five[16] or ten years[12]. As mortality rates rise with age – for instance an increase of two years between the ages of 70 and 79 is associated with an increase in mortality rate of 20%[5], the observed difference could simply have been due to age differences between infected and non-infected subjects. In order to circumvent this problem, Nordenstam *et al.* followed up a large cohort of seventy-year-olds who were stratified into groups with a two-month age range, and was unable to substantiate Dontas *et al.* and Souranders and Kasanen's findings[5]. Furthermore, in the study by Sourander and

Kasanen, patients were classified on the basis of only one MSSU[16]. A single MSSU is frequently inaccurate, being associated with high false positive rates in old age[23]. Thus, it is likely that many patients were erroneously categorized as having UTI.

In addition, all the studies had a major flaw, in that subjects were initially classified as either bacteriuric or abacteriuric and this status could not subsequently be changed. As has already been noted, the number of elderly patients affected by UTI steadily rises with time, but the overall prevalence remains fairly static[11,16,17]. Thus, in many instances, UTIs would have resolved, or have arisen in previously unaffected subjects. This flux may have obscured any differences between the groups. If, however, only patients with persistently sterile or infected urine had been included, perhaps more clear-cut results would have emerged. Dontas *et al.* subsequently discounted the data for patients with intermittent bacteriuria, and, in fact, found no differ-ence in mortality rates. The numbers in each group – 10 and 25 respectively – were too small to draw valid conclusions[19].

In all these studies, the number of bacteriuric subjects was relatively small. As mortality rates in old age are high already, it is likely that only a major effect of UTI on mortality rates could have been detected.

The literature, therefore, does not provide convincing evidence that, in old age, UTI shortens life expectancy. Nevertheless, it is likely that UTI is associated with excess mortality in the elderly[19,61]. Support for this comes from the much larger study of Evans *et al.* where over a twelve- to fifteen-year follow-up period mortality rates amongst adult women with UTI were 1.5 times greater than for unaffected women[62].

Significantly, none of these studies reported an excess of deaths from septicaemia or renal failure amongst subjects with UTI. Hence, there is little evidence to suggest that UTI is a direct cause of excess mortality. It is much more likely that UTIs are associated with factors which do adversely affect mortality rates, but what these might be is not yet known.

MORBIDITY

Just as the effect of UTI on life expectancy in the elderly is the subject of controversy, so too is its relationship with morbidity. As has been discussed, UTI seldom causes dysuria, and there is little evidence to suggest that simple UTI results in problems, such as confusion, falls, incontinence, and 'failure to thrive'[47]. In this section, the relationship between UTI and renal function, hypertension and propensity to bacteraemia are discussed.

Effect on renal function

Long-term studies of adults have not detected a relationship between declining renal function (when measured crudely by sequential serum creatinine levels) and simple UTI[63]. There is no reason to suggest that this should not also be the case in the elderly, and there are several reports which support such a view, as serum creatinine levels appear to be unaffected by UTI[28,46]. Moreover, Freeman et al.'s prospective study found no deterioration of renal function in mainly elderly males with recurrent UTI, although follow up was only 2 years[58]. Nevertheless, when more subtle observations were made, as in the small studies by Marketos et al. and Dontas et al., an accelerated decline in renal function was demonstrated in association with UTI[12,64]. Marketos et al. found that renal blood flow declined more rapidly in elderly patients with UTI, and Dontas followed 12 such patients over two years and found a 20% reduction in creatinine clearance, as opposed to 5% in age-matched controls. Initial creatinine clearances were, however, significantly lower in the bacteriuric group and it may be that, rather than UTI affecting renal blood flow, it is impaired renal blood flow which predisposes to infection.

In old age[7], as at younger ages[65], UTI may be associated with impaired tubular concentrating capacity. The long-term significance of such changes is likely to be benign; Zinner and Kass found no decline in creatinine clearance over a 14-year period in women with tubular concentrating abnormalities secondary to UTI[66].

Certainly, as has already been discussed, there is little evidence that persistent UTI causes renal failure in the elderly. It has been suggested that these more subtle alterations in renal function reduce the ability of elderly patients to counteract changes brought about by unrelated disease, and, in that way, contribute to morbidity and mortality[7]. There is, however, little evidence to support such conjecture.

Hypertension

If hypertension were shown to result from UTI in the elderly, this might provide an explanation for the increased mortality rates which some workers have reported in association with UTI. In younger adults, there does appear to be an increased incidence of hypertension amongst patients with UTI[67], and UTI is found more often in hypertensive subjects[68]. In the healthy aged, this does not seem to be the case, although a high incidence in hypertension has been reported in chronically ill bed-ridden elderly subjects with UTI[69]. From a therapeutic point of view, however, there is no evidence that treating occult UTI results in a fall in blood pressure[70].

Bacteraemia

Given that UTI is common in old age, what proportion of affected patients will develop bacteraemia? Large prospective studies, both in the community and in hospital, suggest that UTI seldom causes bacteraemia in non-catheterized elderly subjects[12,16,18]. Nevertheless, the urinary tract is the commonest source of bacteraemia in old age, both in hospitalized patients and in those admitted from the community[71-73], and many will have undergone catheterization[72,74]. In one study of elderly bacteraemic in-patients, 17% had a source of infection in the urinary tract, and, of these patients, 70% had been catheterized[72]. From that study, it was estimated that approximately 3% of elderly catheterized in-patients will develop bacteraemia.

Many elderly patients do not present with classical clinical features of acute pyelonephritis, such as loin pain and dysuria, and often fail to mount a leucocytosis. Moreover, altered levels of consciousness and pre-eminent gastrointestinal and respiratory symptoms may further divert attention from the urinary tract[74]. Furthermore, as UTI is so widespread in old age, especially amongst those with catheters, the urinary tract should not be accepted as the source of bacteraemia unless the same organism is grown from simultaneous blood and urine cultures. As single blood cultures are often sterile, several samples should be taken[74].

E. coli is the organism isolated most frequently from non-catheterized patients; *Proteus mirabilis, Pseudomonas aeruginosa,* and *Klebsiella* spp are uncommon[74]. For catheterized subjects, although *E. coli* is still the commonest single pathogen, other enterobacteria are found more often[74].

Radiological assessment is warranted, especially for patients without catheters, as a significant proportion will have structural abnormalities, such as urinary obstruction, calculus disease, and peri-nephric abscesses, which may be amenable to surgery[75].This is especially the case when patients remain febrile despite appropriate antibiotics[54]. Initial therapy should be with antibiotics active against the enterobacteria, including *Pseudomonas aeruginosa*. An amino-glycoside combined with a third-generation cephalosporin are therefore appropriate antibiotics until antimicrobial sensitivities are available.

The prognosis varies according to whether bacteraemia develops at home or in hospital. If it develops at home, the prognosis is good[73]. Conversely, mortality rates may be as high as 30% amongst cathet-erized in-patients who develop bacteraemia secondary to UTI[72]. Such high mortality rates, however, seem to be mainly limited to patients with an already poor prognosis from unrelated diseases[72,73]. Never-theless, the studies of Platt *et al.* suggested that mortality rates could be reduced by up to one-half amongst such high-risk patients by using sealed catheter collecting systems or prescribing antibiotics during catheterization[76,77].

There is, therefore, little evidence that the non-catheterized elderly patient with UTI is at particular risk of developing bacteraemia. If bacteraemia does occur, the prognosis is generally good. Catheterized in-patients are at considerable risk of bacteraemia, and, therefore, may benefit from the use of sealed catheter systems or antibiotics during catheterization.

MANAGEMENT

Should UTI in old age be treated? As the elderly are a heterogeneous group, there is no all-encompassing answer to this question. What emerges from the literature is that, although there are a few patients who do benefit from therapy, there is little evidence that the great majority warrant treatment and they may even be harmed by antibiotic side effects. In order to justify therapy, it must be shown that the elderly are at risk from UTI, that therapy is effective, and can confer benefit. As has been discussed, there is little evidence, apart from Platt et al.'s study of catheterized hospital in-patients, to suggest that UTI causes excess mortality[76,77]. Moreover, in the study by Nicolle et al. of non-catheterized males in long-term care, mortality rates were not altered by therapy, and the response to treatment was disappointing[3]. In addition, Boscia et al.'s study suggested that therapy has no effect on general well being[47]. Although GFR and renal blood flow fall more rapidly in patients with UTI, it is unknown whether treatment reverses such trends[12,64].

Given the extensive nature of UTI in old age, treating all affected patients would involve considerable expense. It has been estimated that about one-third of antibiotics used in geriatric wards are for UTI. The elderly are not only at increased risk of side effects from antibiotics but such liberal use encourages resistance to broad-spectrum antibiotics and increases the incidence of Pseudomonas aeruginosa infections[49,78]. Moreover, many UTIs are transient and resolve without recourse to therapy[4,11].

There are, therefore, compelling arguments for not treating all UTIs, especially occult ones. In certain circumstances, of course, antibiotics are warranted. Patients with renal impairment should be considered for treatment. Those with urinary symptoms should receive therapy; although, in the majority, such symptoms are secondary to age-related anatomical changes, there are some in whom the symptoms will resolve with treatment[24]. A trial of therapy has also been advocated for patients who are deteriorating physically and intellectually[79], but the response has been generally disappointing. Where there is evidence of calculus disease, and urea-splitting organisms are grown, or if there is evidence of urological obstruction and the patient is unsuitable for surgery, therapy should be given, as it should be for immunosuppressed patients or those with prosthetic joints, heart valve disease and pacemakers[80]. Hospitalized patients undergoing bladder catheterization should also be treated, as the study of Platt *et al.* demonstrated a striking reduction in mortality rates by using sealed catheter connection systems or antibiotics[77].

TREATMENT

When appropriate antibiotics are prescribed, the majority of MSSUs will become sterile[3,81-83]. In the elderly, short courses of antibiotics appear to be more effective than single-dose or one-day treatments[81-83]. Short courses (less than five days) are preferable because compliance is increased – which is especially relevant in the elderly, and because the chances of side effects and drug interactions are reduced. For patients whose symptoms are controlled by infrequent discrete courses of antibiotics, long-term therapy is not required. In some, however, infection will rapidly recur with the same organism. This is termed relapse and occurs because the organism has not been eradicated. The causes of relapse are not well defined in elderly women, but, in men, data derived from fluorescent antibody coating of bacteria tests indicate that, in most instances of relapse, tissue invasion has occurred[57]. Relapses in males are often associated with urinary obstruction or with underlying structural abnormalities in the urinary tract, such as calculus disease, renal scars and prostatic disease, not readily penetrated by antibiotics[58,84]. In addition relapse may be due to faecal or urinary incontinence causing perineal contamination. Treatment of incontinence is more effective in reducing the incidence of bacterial relapse than antibiotic therapy (which is almost invariably unsuccessful) in such patients[24,78].

Rapid relapse should prompt investigations to define underlying urological abnormalities, although these are often amenable only to surgery. Hence, the vigour of subsequent investigations will depend on the underlying health of the patient.

In males, the seat of recurrent infection is often the prostate gland, as a consequence of either chronic prostatitis or prostatic microcalculi. Chronic prostatitis is symptomless and not visible on IVP unless associated with prostatic hypertrophy, and plain X-ray often fails to detect prostatic calculi[85]. Infection may be localized to the prostate using the method described by Meares and Stamey[86]. Using this method, a ten-fold rise in colony-forming units in the urine following prostatic massage generally indicates a source of infection within the prostate. Trimethoprim is one of the few antibiotics active against Gram-negative organisms which can achieve therapeutic levels within the prostate[85]. Even with trimethoprim, the response is often poor[10,57]. In one study, only six of nineteen patients were cured by three months of continuous trimethoprim therapy, and, in another, only three of six patients were cured by four months treatment[10]. Prostatic calculi exacerbate the problem, as infected calculi are not sterilized by antimicrobial treatment[85]. Long-term treatment with 100 mg nitrofurantoin daily may render patients free of symptoms[85], and, because of limited exposure of the organism to nitrofurantoin, resistance is not often a problem[10]. Such treatment, however, only prolongs the intervals between relapse and is not curative[58].

Surgery may be considered for men with recurrent symptomatic UTIs who fail to respond to antibiotics. However, because the peripheral prostate often contains foci of infection, sometimes only recourse to radical prostatectomy results in a cure. Many elderly men may not be fit for such surgery, which also carries a significant risk of urinary incontinence.

The efficacy of prophylactic antibiotic treatment for elderly females is not well defined. Urinary antiseptics, such as nitrofurantoin after initial urine sterilization have proved of benefit in long-stay geriatric patients[24].

Antibiotics

The incidence of drug toxicity and side effects is increased in old age[87,88]. Lean body mass decreases with age; hence, if lipid-insoluble drugs, such as aminoglycosides, are administered on a milligram per kilogram basis, toxicity can result from even standard doses. Furthermore, the elderly, because of concomitant drug therapy, are at greater risk of drug interactions.

The main antibiotics used for UTIs are the penicillins, trimethoprim, sulphonamides, nitrofurantoin, nalidixic acid, and second-generation cephalosporins. Because most UTIs are due to gut-derived commensals, drugs which alter colonic flora will rapidly select resistant pathogens amongst the enterobacteria, which are capable of acquiring plasmid transferred resistance. This problem is most marked with penicillins but also occurs to a lesser extent with trimethoprim, sulphonamides, cephalosporins and nalidixic acid[34].

Nitrofurantoin is almost totally absorbed in the upper gastro-intestinal tract and thus is a useful drug, as resistance rates remain low even with long-term therapy. It can be poorly tolerated in the elderly and is contraindicated in the presence of renal impairment because of the risks of polyneuropathy, and, when prescribed for long periods, can cause pulmonary fibrosis[79].

Trimethroprim–sulphonamide combinations may exacerbate bor-derline folate deficiencies and may also potentiate the actions of tolbutamide and warfarin and occasionally induce Stevens–Johnson syndrome[79]. Nalidixic acid can also potentiate the effects of warfarin, and cephalosporins and frusemide may enhance the nephrotoxicity of aminoglycosides[89].

Oestrogen therapy

After the menopause, low oestrogen levels probably predispose to recurrent UTIs. Two studies have reported successful treatment of symptomatic UTI using continuous low-dose intravaginal oestrogen. Patients treated had recurrent symptomatic UTI despite repeated courses of antibiotics[32,90]. After initial sterilization of urine with a short course of antibiotics, intravaginal oestrogen cream was commenced. Most patients became asymptomatic thereafter, and this was main-tained by approximately twice-weekly applications of cream con-taining 1–2 mg oestrogen.

CONCLUSION

The significance of UTI in old age is not known. It is difficult to base realistic conclusions on the current literature, as all published studies have diagnosed UTI on the criterion of 10^5 or more colony-forming units per ml of urine. Whether this criterion is applicable to the elderly (or many other patient groups) is debatable. It has been suggested that only a large multicentre collaborative project could produce valid conclusions because of the large numbers of patients required to produce statistically meaningful results. However, before embarking on such a project, specific diagnostic criteria would have to be devised which were applicable to the elderly. Such a project would involve considerable time and expense and is unlikely to be performed. Nevertheless, UTI is a common occurrence in old age. The current literature provides little evidence to suggest that, in the majority, it has a detrimental affect on health. It does, however, suggest that certain groups of patients are at risk from UTI and so should be treated.

ACKNOWLEDGEMENT

I am grateful to Mrs Fiona Ashby for preparing this manuscript.

REFERENCES

1. Kass, E. H. (1956). Asymptomatic infection of the urinary tract. *Trans. Assoc. Am. Physicians,* **69,** 59
2. Alling, B., Brandberg, A., Seeberg, S. and Svanburg, A. (1973). Aerobic and anaerobic microbial flora in the urinary tract of geriatric patients during longterm care. *J. Infect. Dis.,* **127,** 34–39
3. Nicolle, L. E., Bjornson, J., Harding, G. K. and MacDonell, J. A. (1983). Bacteriuria in elderly institutionalized men. *N. Engl. J. Med.,* **309,** 420–45.
4. Wolfson, S. A., Kalmanson, G. M., Rubini, M. E. and Guze, L. S. (1965). Epidemiology of bacteriuria in a predominantly geriatric male population. *Am. J. Med. Sci.,* **250,** 168–173
5. Nordenstam, G. R., Brandberg, C. A., Oden, A. S., Svanborg Eden, C. M. and Svanbord, A. 1986). Bacteriuria and mortality in an elderly population. *N. Engl. J. Med.,* **314,** 1152–1156
6. Dontas, A. S., Paraskaki, I., Petrikkos, G. and Giamarellou, H. (1987). Diuresis bacteriuria in physically dependent elderly women. *Age Ageing,* **16,** 215–220
7. Dontas, A. S. (1984). Urinary tract infections and their implications. In Brocklehurst, J. C. (ed.) *Urology in the Elderly,* pp. 162–195. (Edinburgh: Churchill-Livingston)
8. Sourander, L. B. (1966). Urinary tract infection in the aged – an epidemiological study. *Ann. Med. Intern. Fenniae,* **55** (Suppl. 45), 7–55
9. Brocklehurst, J. C., Dillane, J. B., Griffiths, L. and Fry, J. (1968). The prevalence

and symptomatology of urinary infection in an aged population. *Gerontol. Clin.,* **10,** 242–253

10. Mayer, T. R. (1980). Urinary tract infection in the elderly: How to select treatment. *Geriatrics,* **35** (March), 67–77

11. Boscia, J. A., Kobasa, W. D., Knight, R. A., Abrutyn, E., Levison, M. E. and Kaye, D. (1986). Epidemiology of bacteriuria in an elderly ambulatory population. *Am. J. Med.,* **80,** 208–214

12. Dontas, A. S., Kasviki-Charvati, P., Papanayiotou, P. C. and Marketos, S. G. (1981). Bacteriuria and survival in old age. *N. Engl. J. Med.,* **304,** 939–943

13. Walkey, F. A., Judge, T. G., Thompson, J. and Sarkari, N. B. (1967). Incidence of urinary infection in the elderly. *Scot. Med. J.,* **12,** 411–414

14. Sourander, L. B., Ruikka, I. and Gronroos, M. (1965). Correlation between urinary tract infection, prolapse conditions and function of the bladder in aged female hospital patients. *Gerontol. Clin.,* **7,** 179–184

15. Gibson, I. J. M. and Pritchard, J. G. (1965). Screen investigation of the elderly. *Gerontol. Clin.,* **7,** 330–336

16. Sourander, L. B. and Kasanen, A. (1972). 5-year follow-up of bacteriuria in the aged. *Gerontol. Clin.,* **14,** 274–281

17. Kasviki-Charvati, P., Drolette-Kefakis, B., Papanayiotou, P, C. and Dontas, A. S. (1982). Turnover of bacteriuria in old age. *Age Ageing,* **11,** 169–174

18. Nicolle, L. E., Henderson, E., Bjornson, J., McIntyre, M. Harding, G. K. and MacDonell, J. A. (1987). Association of bacteriuria with resident characteristics and survival in elderly institutionalised men. *Ann. Intern. Med.,* **106,** 682–686

19. Dontas, A. S, (1986). Urinary tract infection in old age. In Asscher, A. W. and Brumfitt, W. (eds.) *Microbial Diseases in Nephrology,* p. 287. (Chichester: John Wiley and Sons)

20. Shock, N. W. (1962). The physiology of ageing: *Sci. Am.,* **206,** 100–110

21. Gardiner, I. A. (1980). The effects of ageing on susceptibility to infection. *Rev. Infect. Dis.,* **2,** 801–80

22. Kaye, D. (1980). Urinary tract infection in the elderly. *Bull. N. Y. Acad. Med.,* **56,** 209–220

23. Lye, M. (1978). Defining and treating urinary infections. *Geriatrics,* **33** (3), 71–77

24. Brocklehurst, J. C., Bee, P., Jones, D. and Palmer, M. K. (1977). Bacteriuria in geriatric hospital patients: its correlates and management. *Age Ageing,* **6,** 240–245

25. Bentzen, A. and Vejlsgaard, R. (1980). Asymptomatic bacteriuria in elderly subjects. *Danish Med. Bull.,* **27,** 101–105

26. Stamey, T. A. (1975). The role of vaginal colonization with enterobacteriaceae in recurrent urinary tract infection. *J. Urol.,* **113,** 214–217

27. Cox, C. E., Lacy, S. S. and Hinman, F. (1968). The urethra and its relationship to urinary tract infection. ii. The urethral flora of the female with recurrent urinary tract infection. *J. Urol.* **99,** 632–635

28. Heinamaki, D., Haavisto, M., Mattila, K. and Rajala, S. (1984). Urinary characteristics and infection in the very aged. *Gerontology,* **30,** 403–407

29. Dymock, S. (1973). In Brocklehurst, J. C. (ed.) *Textbook of Geriatric Medicine and Gerontology,* p. 309. (Edinburgh: Churchill Livingstone)

30. Parvinen, M., Sourander, L. B. and Vourinen, P. (1965). Cystographic studies of old women. *Gerontol. Clin.,* **7,** 343–347

31. Brocklehurst, J. C. and Dillane, J. B. (1966). Studies of the female bladder in old age. 1: Cystometograms in non-incontinent women. *Gerontol. Clin.*, **8**, 285–305
32. Parsons, C. L. and Schmidt, J. D. (1982). Control of recurrent lower urinary tract infection in the post-menopausal woman. *J. Urol.*, **128**, 1224–1226
33. Stamey, T. S. and Timothy, M. M. (1975). Studies of introital colonization in women with recurrent urinary tract infection: The role of vaginal pH. *J. Urol.*, **114**, 261–263
34. Mulholland, S. G. (1986). Controversies in management of urinary tract infection. *Urology*, **17**, 2, suppl. 3–8
35. Kunin, C. M. and McCormick, R. C. (1968). An epidemiological study of bacteriuria and hypertension among nuns and working women. *N. Engl. J. Med.*, **278**, 635–642
36. Reid, G., Zorzitto, M. L., Bruce, A. W., Jewett, M. A. S., Chan, R. C. Y. and Casterton, J. W. (1984). Pathogenesis of urinary tract infection in the elderly. The role of bacterial adherence to uroepithelial cells. *Curr. Microbiol.*, **11**, 67–72
37. Sobel, J. D. and Muller, G. (1984). Pathogenesis of bacteriuria in elderly women: The role of *Escherichia coli* adherence to vaginal epithelial cells. *J. Gerontol.*, **39** (6), 682–685
38. Sobel, J. D. and Kaye, D. (1985). Reduced uromucoid excretion in the elderly. *J. Infect. Dis.*, **152**, 653
39. Jaffe, J. W. (1978). Common lower urinary tract problems on older persons. In Reicke, W. (ed.) *Clinical Aspects of Ageing*, p. 228. (Baltimore: Williams and Wilkins Co.)
40. Meares, E. M. (1975). Prostatitis: a review. *Urol. Clin. N. Am.*, **2**, 3–27
41. Anderson, R. U. (1986). Urinary tract infections in compromised hosts. *Urol. Clin. N. Am.*, **13**, 4, 752–753
42. Gladstone, J. L. and Friedman, S. A. (1971). Bacteriuria on the aged: A study of its prevalence and predisposing factors in a chronically ill population. *J. Urol.*, 745–749
43. Hirsh, D. D., Fainstein, V. and Musher, D. M. (1979). Do condom catheter collecting systems cause urinary tract infection? *J. Am. Med. Assoc.*, **242**, 340–341
44. Johnson, E. T. (1983). The condom catheter: urinary tract infection and other complications. *South. Med. J.*, **76**, 579–582
45. Fierer, J. and Ekstrom, M. (1983). An outbreak of Providencia stuartti urinary tract infection – Patients with condom catheters are a reservoir of infection. *South. Med. J.*, **76**, 579–582
46. Akhtar, A. J., Andrews, G. R., Caird, F. I. and Fallon, R. J. (1972). Urinary tract infection in the elderly: a population study. *Age Ageing*, **1**, 48–54
47. Boscia, J. A., Kobasa, W. D., Abrutyn, E., Levison, M. E., Kaplan, A. M. and Kaye, D. (1986). Lack of association between bacteriuria and symptoms in the elderly. *Am. J. Med.*, **81**, 979–982
48. Norman, D. C., Castle, S. C. and Cantrell, M. (1987). Infections in the nursing home. *J. Am. Geriatr. Soc.*, **35**, 796–805
49. Bendall, M. J. (1984). A review of urinary tract infection in the elderly. *J. Antimicrob. Chemother.*, **13** (suppl B), 69–78
50. Choudbury, S. L. and Brocklehurst, J. C. (1987). Urinary tract infection in old age. In Macias-Nunez, J. F. and Cameron, J. S. (eds) *Renal Function and Disease in the Elderly*, pp. 254–281. (London: Butterworths)

51. Moore-Smith, B. (1974). The treatment of urinary tract infections in elderly women. *Mod. Geriatr.*, **4**, 408–413.
52. Andriole, V. T. (1972). Diagnosis of urinary tract infection by culture. In Kaye, D. (ed.) *Urinary tract Infection and Management*, p. 37. (St Louis: CV Mosby Co.)
53. Gleckman, R. and Esposito, A. (1979). Sterile pyuria in the elderly. *Am. Fam. Physician*, **19** (6), 109–111
54. Gleckman, R., Blagg, N., Hibert, D. *et al.* (1982). Acute pyelonephritis in the elderly. *South. Med. J.*, **75**, 551–554
55. Suntharalingham, M., Seth, V. and Moore-Smith, B. (1983). Site of urinary tract infection in elderly women admitted to an acute geriatric assessment unit. *Age Ageing*, **12**, 317–322
56. Fairley, K. F., Bon, A. G., Brown, R. B. and Habersberger, P. (1967). Simple test to determine the site of urinary tract infection. *Lancet*, **2**, 427–428
57. Smith, S. W., Jones, S. R., Reed, W. P., Tice, A. D., Deupress, R. H and Kaijser, B. (1979). Recurrent urinary tract infections in men: Characteristics and response to therapy. *Ann. Intern. Med.*, **91**, 544–548
58. Freeman, R. B., McFate-Smith, W. and Richardson, J. A. (1975). Long-term therapy for chronic bacteriuria in men. *Ann. Intern. Med.*, **83**, 133–147
59. Thompson, E. G. and Eastwood, M. R. (1981). Survivorship and senile dementia. *Age Ageing*, **10**, 29–32
60. Kirkland, J. L. and Robinson, J. M. (1981). Bacteriuria and survival in old age. *N. Engl. J. Med.*, **305**, 586
61. Kass, E. H. (1985). Bacteriuria and excess mortality: what should the next steps be? *Rev. Infect. Dis.*, **7** (suppl. 4), S762–S766
62. Evans, D. A., Kass, E. H., Hennekens, C. H. *et al.* (1982). Bacteriuria and subsequent mortality in women. *Lancet*, **1** (8264), 156–158
63. Asscher, A. W., Verrier-Jones, K. and Harber (1986). In Asscher, A. W. and Brumfitt, W. (eds) *Microbial Diseases in Nephrology*, p. 93. (Chichester: John Wiley and Sons)
64. Marketos, S. G., Papanayiotou, P. C. and Dontas, A.S. (1969). Bacteriuria and non-obstructive renovascular disease in old age. *J. Gerontol.*, **24**, 33–36
65. Clarke, H., Roland, A. R., Cutler, R. E. and Turk, M. (1969). The correlation between site of infections and maximal concentrating ability in bacteriuria. *J. Infect. Dis.*, **120**, 47–51
66. Zinner, S. H. and Kass, E. H. (1971). Longterm (10–14 years) follow-up of bacteriuria in pregnancy. *N. Engl. J. Med.*, **285**, 820–827
67. Kass, E. H., Miall, W. E. and Stewart, K. L. (1961). Relationship of bacteriuria to hypertension; an epidemiological study. *J. Clin. Invest.*, **40**, 1053
68. Kass, E. H., Miall, W. E., Stewart, K. L. and Rosner, B. (1978). Epidemiological aspects of infections of the urinary tract. In Kass, E. H. and Brumfitt, W. (eds) *Infections of the urinary Tract*, pp. 1–7: (Chicago: University of Chicago Press)
69. Marketos, S. G., Dontas, A. S., Papanayiotou, F. and Economou, P. (1970). Bacteriuria and hypertension in old age. *Geriatrics*, **25**, 136–147
70. Asscher, A. W. (1980). *The Challenge of Urinary Tract Infections*, p. 71. (London: Academic Press)
71. Esposito, A. L., Gleckman, R. A., Crom, S., Crawley, M., Mcabe, F. and Drapkin, M. S. (1980). Community acquired bacteraemia in the elderly: Analysis of one hundred consecutive episodes. *J. Am. Geriatr. Soc.*, **28**, 315–319

72. Bryan, C. S. and Reynolds, K. L. (1984). Hospital acquired bacteremic urinary tract infection: epidemiology and outcome. *J. Urol.*, **132,** 494–497
73. Bryan, C. S. and Reynolds, K. L. (1984). Community acquired bacteremic urinary tract infection: epidemiology and outcome. *J. Urol.*, **132,** 490–494
74. Gleckman, R., Blagg, N., Hibert, D. *et al.* (1982). Community-acquired bacteremic urosepsis in the elderly patients: A prospective study of 34 consecutive episodes. *J. Urol.*, **128,** 79–81
75. Gleckman, R., Blagg, N., Hibert, D. *et al.* (1982). Symptomatic pyelonephritis in elderly men. *J. Am. Geriatr. Soc.*, **30** (11), 690–693
76. Platt, R., Polk, B. F., Murdock, B. and Rosner, B. (1982). Mortality associated with nosocomial urinary tract infection. *N. Engl. J. Med.*, **307,** 637–642
77. Platt, R., Polk, B. F., Murdock, B. and Rosner, B. (1983). Reduction in mortality associated with nosocomial urinary tract infection. *Lancet,* **1,** 893–897
78. Alling, B., Brandberg, A., Seeberg, S. and Svanburg, A. (1975). Effect of consecutive antibacterial therapy on bacteria in hospitalised geriatric patients. *Scand. J. Infect. Dis.,* **7,** 201–207
79. Sourander, L. B. and Rowe, J. W. (1985). The genito-urinary system – the ageing kidney. In Brocklehurst, J. C. (ed.) *Textbook of Geriatrics and Gerontology,* pp. 609–625. (Edinburgh: Churchill-Livingstone)
80. Shortcliffe, L. M. D. (1986). Asymptomatic bacteriuria: Should it be treated. *Urology Suppl.,* **27,** S19–25
81. Boscia, J. A., Kobasa, W. D., Knight, R. A., Abrutyn, E., Levison, M. E. and Kaye, D. (1987). Therapy vs no therapy for bacteriuria in elderly ambulatory non-hospitalised women. *J. Am. Med. Assoc.*, **257,** 1067–1071
82. Renneberg, J. and Paserregaard, A. (1984). Single-day treatment with trimethoprim for asymptomatic bacteriuria in the elderly patient. *J. Urol.*, **132,** 934–935
83. Lacey, R. W., Simpson, M. H. C., Lord, V. L., Fawcett, C., Bulton, E. S., Laxton, D. E. A. and Trotter, I. S. (1981). Comparison of single dose trimethoprim with a five day course for the treatment of urinary tract infections in the elderly. *Age Ageing,* **10,** 179–185
84. Gleckman, R. Crowley, M. and Natsios, G. A. (1979), Therapy of recurrent invasive urinary tract infection. *N. Engl. J. Med.,* **301,** 878–880
85. Meares, E. M. Jr and Barbalias, G.A. (1983). Prostatitis: Bacterial, non-bacterial and prostatodynia. *Semin. Urol.,* **1,** 146–154
86. Meares, E. M. and Stamey, T. A. (1968). Bacteriologic localisation patterns in bacterial prostatitis and urethritis. *Invest. Urol.,* **5,** 492–518
87. Grieco, M. H. (1980). Use of antibiotics in the elderly. *Bull. N.Y. Acad. Med.,* **56,** 197–208
88. Moellering, R. C. (1978). Factors influencing the clinical use of antimicrobial agents in elderly patients. *Geriatrics,* **33,** 83–91
89. Gleckman, R. A. and Esposito, A. L. (1980). Antibiotics in the elderly: skating on therapeutic thin ice. *Geriatrics,* **35,** 26–37
90. Privette, M., Cade, R., Petersen, J. and Mars, D. (1988). Prevention of recurrent urinary tract infection in postmenopausal women. *Nephron,* **50,** 24–27
91. Medical Research Council Bacteriuria Committee (1979). Recommended Terminology of urinary tract infection. *Br. Med. J.,* **2,** 717–719
92. Asscher, A. W. (1980). *The Challenge of Urinary Tract Infections*, p. 8. (London: Academic Press)

4

UROLOGICAL PROBLEMS

L. E. F. MOFFAT AND S. McCLINTON

This chapter will deal with urological problems as they present to the urologist in roughly chronological order, from urinary tract infection (UTI) in childhood but excluding UTI in the elderly (Chapter 3). Problems associated with treatment will also be discussed, including catheter management, the ileal loop and, finally, antibiotic prophylaxis during urinary tract surgery.

UTI IN CHILDHOOD

It is now recognized that much of the renal scarring seen in the older child will have occurred within the first year or two of life and new scars are seldom seen after the age of five years[1]. It is important that unexplained pyrexias should be investigated by midstream specimens of urine (MSSU) and, if necessary, by bladder aspiration. Ultrasound is now used by many as a first line in imaging investigation in youngsters. All cases of urinary obstruction require appropriate correction. Surgical correction of reflux is now required much less often since antibiotics can control infection in approximately 75% of cases[1]. There has been much controversy over the use of Teflon injected in a subureteric position (the STING procedure)[2]. This partially occludes the ureteric orifice. The technique appears to reduce reflux and the major objection would seem to be uncertainty over the long-term effects of the Teflon. The technique can be used at cystoscopy as a day patient and will undoubtedly become more popular.

THE SCHOOLCHILD WITH BACTERIURIA

Schoolchildren are occasionally referred, having been found to have asymptomatic bacteriuria. In schoolgirls, it is rare for the bacteriuria to be sustained, and, where it is not, they may be discharged. The girl with sustained bacteriuria and the schoolboy with one episode of bacteriuria require either ultrasound of their kidneys or an intravenous urogram (IVU). A carbonated drink can be given prior to the IVU as this forms a 'window' through the stomach allowing better definition of the upper tracts. It is wise to cystoscope these patients to rule out remediable problems.

THE WOMAN WITH RECURRENT UTI

Most women will experience pain or discomfort when passing urine at some time during their life. It is often accompanied by urgency and frequency of micturition. For most women, these symptoms are a minor and infrequent annoyance but, for some women, they are recurrent and very debilitating. A minority may also, of course, develop more serious upper tract infections with symptoms of fever, rigors and general malaise. The infection is most commonly due to autoinfection from the faecal flora, particularly *Escherichia coli,* and, in the community, will respond to almost all the broad-spectrum antimicrobial agents available. However, as the symptoms and treatment become recurrent, resistant strains emerge and other Gram-negative infections develop. Urinary antiseptics have a place. Basic advice is often appreciated. The woman should be instructed to 'work away' from her perineum on cleaning herself after defaecation, to avoid nylon underwear, and to empty her bladder after sexual intercourse. A few patients may require to be issued with antibiotic tablets to be taken after intercourse (or indeed before, if feasible).

Investigations should include either an IVU or ultrasound of the kidneys and bladder. Cystourethroscopy may give diagnostic information and urethral overdilatation can give symptomatic relief. Only a small proportion of patients have a significant bladder urinary residue and the mechanism may be 'milking' of the urethral glands. In resistant cases, prophylactic antibiotics may be required. A single daily dose of trimethoprim, taken at night, may be effective.

UTI IN PREGNANCY

Urologists see relatively few pregnant women with UTI's as most are treated by the obstetrician or the general practitioner. Those who are referred to the urologist are usually the more serious cases. The incidence of UTI in pregnant women is within the range known to exist in non-pregnant women of childbearing age[3] and is reported[4] as being between 4–7%. Forty per cent of patients with untreated UTIs will go on to develop symptomatic acute pyelonephritis[3], particularly in the third trimester. For this reason, all pregnant women require to be screened for asymptomatic bacteriuria at their first prenatal visit. Of those who have a positive bacteriuria at first screening 20–30% are likely to develop recurrent UTIs throughout their pregnancy. Treatment should aim at eliminating bacteria from the urinary tract and, because recurrent infection is common, MSSUs should be obtained throughout pregnancy. There is no convincing data to date of any adverse consequences of UTIs on the fetus although a higher rate of premature labour has been reported[5]. Anatomical changes which occur during pregnancy include:

(a) Dilatation of the calyces, renal pelvis and ureter which is most marked in the third trimester, and
(b) Reduced peristaltic activity.

These changes are thought to be due both to a mechanical effect of the pregnancy and to the action of progesterone-like hormones produced during the pregnancy. It should also be remembered that the bladder becomes an abdominal organ during pregnancy. All these changes are most marked in the third trimester and this is when severe infections are most likely.

Women are usually referred to the urologist if they fail to improve symptomatically despite the use of appropriate antibiotics or if the urine cultures show recurrence of bacteriuria after initial clearance on appropriate treatment. Often, these are patients who have an abnormality of their renal tracts and they require full urological investigation and occasionally surgical intervention.

PYELONEPHRITIS

Pyelonephritis is an infection of the renal substance and it is of no surprise that the symptoms are more severe than those of uncomplicated UTI. Classically, the patient may complain of fever, chills and flank pain with associated prostration and variable gastrointestinal symptoms due to ileus. Only half of these patients may have lower urinary tract symptoms. Presentation is more obscure in the elderly and in the neonate. The organisms are usually Enterobacteriaceae, of which *Escherichia coli* is the main offender. The severity of the disease is modified by predisposing causes, of which ureteric obstruction, renal stone and vesico-ureteric reflux are the main urological causes. The disease may be much more aggressive in the diabetic and in the immunosuppressed patient. Elderly patients may not have good immune responses and are less able to tolerate this condition.

An intense inflammatory response develops in the kidney and can lead to scarring with variable loss of renal function. The presence of obstruction exacerbates renal destruction but it is principally during the first three years of life that this risk is greatest. The juvenile kidney is presumably more susceptible to infection and infection is often unrecognized in this age group. Treatment should be given promptly in the form of intravenous antibiotics, such as third-generation penicillins or cephalosporins, and should be initiated once urine and blood cultures have been obtained. It is not necessary to await results since treatment can be instituted on a 'best guess basis'[6] and modified subsequently in the light of reported antibiotic sensitivity.

Failure of response should suggest the presence of a renal or perinephric abscess. This is readily detected on ultrasound and may be drained percutaneously at the same procedure. It is only if the pus is too inspissated that surgical drainage at open operation is required. A sample of the pus can be sent for Gram-stain immediately and also for culture. It is better to send as much pus as possible in a universal container rather than on a swab. Pus may drain into the urinary tract and pyonephrosis may result. It is imperative that the kidney be drained to allow any urine to be excreted and percutaneous drainage is usually appropriate. Unless the clinical condition of the patient is deteriorating, it is wise to be as conservative as possible since useful renal function may be recovered. It is rare nowadays to require immediate surgical intervention to remove the kidney or to take out any obstructing stone, given that adequate drainage has been established and that appropriate antibiotics have been given. The condition of emphysematous pyelonephritis may be an exception. Gas in the renal tissues is only found in diabetics and carries a high mortality. Nephrectomy under antibiotic cover is indicated. The presence of gas in the collecting system is not confined to diabetics and a more conservative approach would normally be indicated[7].

THE MAN WITH UTI

In most urological units in the UK, the appearance of one UTI is taken as an indication that urological investigation is required. The upper tracts should be imaged by ultrasound or IVU. It would be considered as necessary in most units to perform a cystoscopy. In the young man, a mild urethral stricture may be found and urethrotomy may abolish further infection. In the older man, the predisposing cause may be an enlarged prostate. In the absence of symptoms or signs of urinary hold-up, surveillance may be the best policy. Prostatectomy may be indicated because of obstructive symptoms, and, although UTIs may be reduced in frequency, or even abolished, it is important that the patient is not persuaded into operation on the grounds of abolition of infection, since he and his surgeon may be disappointed.

SEXUALLY TRANSMITTED DISEASE (STD)

The sexually transmitted diseases comprise a broad spectrum of conditions caused by spirochaetes, bacteria, viruses, chlamydia, mycoplasma, protozoa, fungi and parasites. These are normally looked after by the approximately 180 consultants and 200 departments of genitourinary medicine within the National Health Service[8]. Ignorance of the sexually transmitted diseases and their prevention is still widespread[9] although publicity due to the AIDS epidemic should help change this. Indeed, the declining incidence of gonorrhoea in London may be related to worries about the AIDS virus[10]. A recent survey, however, shows that, despite government media campaigns, dangerous sexual attitudes and behaviour continued, and people still remain uncertain of the mechanism of infection[11]. These conditions are best dealt with by specialists in genitourinary medicine who have access to special collection facilities for urethral swabs; their advice should be sought whenever appropriate.

UROLOGICAL TUBERCULOSIS

The incidence of genitourinary tuberculosis in the UK has been steadily declining in line with the decrease in pulmonary tuberculosis. However, it is still a serious disease with potentially catastrophic consequences if it is left untreated. Between 8–10% of people with pulmonary tuberculosis will develop renal tuberculosis due to metastatic spread of organisms through the blood stream. The lag phase between pulmonary infection and renal infection may be from 2 to 20 years (average 8 years)[12]. It is twice as common in men as in women and the majority are in the 20–40 year age group.

The initial presentation is with painless urinary frequency which does not respond to standard antibiotic therapy. Micturition may become painful if secondary infection supervenes. The urine is initially sterile and may, or may not, contain pus cells and red cells. There is often a past history of previous tuberculous infection at a younger age. Diagnosis is based on isolating the tubercle bacillus from the urine after all antibiotics have been stopped for at least a week. At least three early-morning specimens of urine (EMSU), and preferably five[13], should be collected and innoculated on to special growth medium. Positive cultures should have sensitivity testing performed against the standard antituberculous drugs.

Further investigations include routine blood studies and an ESR, which is a useful guide to response to therapy. Radiological studies include chest X-ray and an IVU. Endoscopy of the urinary tract may be performed but bladder biopsies should not be taken if there is active tuberculous cystitis since this may lead to tuberculous meningitis.

Treatment for urinary tuberculosis is by short-course chemotherapy (4 months) which has been shown to be as effective as longer courses[14]. This is because the antibiotic levels found in the urine are very high, making short-course therapy effective at sterilizing the urinary tract.

The recommended treatment involves triple therapy for two months, using the standard antituberculous drugs, rifampicin, isoniazid and pyrazinamide, followed by two months of rifampicin and isoniazid alone. Streptomycin may be added to the initial therapy in severe cases[15]. Steroids are not recommended in the initial intensive treatment course but may need to be considered in those cases with ureteric obstruction who do not improve within three weeks of starting chemotherapy. If used, high doses of steroids are required as rifampicin reduces the bioavailability of steroids[16]. Response to treatment is monitored at the end of the four-month treatment course, and at six-monthly intervals thereafter, with three EMSUs. At least one IVU should be obtained during treatment because of the high risk of ureteric stricture formation. Long-term follow up is only recommended for those with calcification in their urinary tract as this may progress after many years[15].

Surgery may be required:

(1) To excise diseased tissue, e.g. nephrectomy for a diseased non-functioning kidney,
(2) To reconstruct a diseased tract, e.g. augmentation procedures for a small contracted bladder, or
(3) More urgently, to relieve ureteric obstruction secondary to stricture formation.

Any surgery should be a planned procedure which, ideally, takes place six weeks after the initiation of chemotherapy. Ureteric strictures occur in 9% of cases[13] and the commonest site is the lower ureter. These may require ureteric reimplantation or simply intubation with a stent. Bladder augmentation is done by enterocystoplasty using either colon or caecum with terminal ileum. Caecum with terminal ileum is especially useful in those cases who also require reimplantation of the ureters[17]. It must be realized that bladder augmentation will not cure enuresis or urinary incontinence.

Prevention of renal tuberculosis will depend on the prevention of pulmonary tuberculosis by contact tracing of infected cases and by the BCG vaccination programmes.

PROSTATITIS

This is a diagnosis which covers a number of problems. Acute bacterial prostatitis is undoubtedly a reality. It can occur in young and old, often, in the latter, in association with prostatic hypertrophy. It would appear to be particularly common in the United States. It usually responds to antibiotics promptly. Co-trimoxazole appears to be particularly effective, perhaps due to its ability to penetrate the acidic environment of the prostate. Reiter's disease, which may lead to diagnostic confusion, is usually distinguished by iritis or by a past history of diarrhoea and sacroiliac signs may be seen on the plain film of an IVU.

Chronic prostatitis is a much more dubious entity[18]. There appear to be no diagnostic pathological changes if biopsy is undertaken. Undoubtedly, at one end of the spectrum of symptoms labelled as chronic prostatitis, is the young man with anxiety of one sort or another. One also sees the businessman who may have committed a sexual indiscretion and has guilt feelings which may often be relieved when the possibility of venereal disease is excluded by investigation. One is then left with a group of men in whom cyclical perineal discomfort with variable dysuria occurs. These patients often respond for a short time to antibiotics, although significant bacteriuria is rarely found. Prostatic massage has its advocates, particularly in the USA, but is far from universally useful. Rotating courses of antibiotics can be useful but they must be used for a number of months to achieve their full effect. A concurrent course of non-steroidal anti-inflammatory agents can be of benefit. Patients diagnosed as having chronic prostatitis are difficult to treat and the urologist is often bereft of any efficacious remedy[19]. Part of the problem may be the way that patients are labelled as suffering from this disease. Undoubtedly, some have psychiatric problems but a convincing explanation for a cyclical illness, often associated with systemic symptoms, has yet to be found. Attempts have been made to isolate a particular pathogen but have been largely unsuccessful. Most recently, Chlamydia has been implicated as a possible agent but the results of treatment have been far from convincing.

UTI AND SEPSIS POST CATHETERIZATION

It is said that over three-quarters of all hospital UTIs are catheter related[20]. It is certainly one of the common conditions seen by urologists. Even if the urine is sterile at the time of catheterization, it will subsequently become infected in most if not all patients. Many infections are difficult, if not impossible, to eradicate once established. Can anything be done to reduce the risk of UTI? Precatheterization antibiotics, on a prophylactic basis, reduce the frequency of bacteriuria but for four days only[21]. Infection gains access, either through the catheter or on the sides of the catheter. The catheter induces a milking action along the sides of the urethra. Urethral secretion is increased and these secretions may not drain adequately. It is important to use as small a catheter as will perform the task required of it. A 16 French catheter is the largest that is normally required for the male bladder. If there are blood clots present, a larger size may be needed and special haematuria catheters are manufactured which have larger orifices at the bulb end to allow clot to be washed out. A three-way catheter with an irrigation channel to keep the bladder free from clot can be useful, especially postoperatively or in the presence of gross haematuria. A siliconized catheter is normally associated with lower rates of infection, but is only necessary when the period of catheterization is expected to be in excess of two weeks.

Infection may be inevitable but there are a number of measures which can be taken to make it less frequent. It is critical that all ward staff exercise care when changing the connections of urinary drainage systems. Hands must be washed in between dealing with each patient. Urine drainage must be of a closed drainage type and steps must be taken to see that it remains so. The drainage bag should have a non-return flutter valve fitted and care should be taken that the bag does not become too full. Gloves should be worn when the bag is changed and urine should be disposed of immediately, and not allowed to lie around a sluice room. Drainage bags should have a rubber port through which urine can be aspirated to provide catheter specimens of urine (CSU). Drainage bags should be below the level of the patient, allowing syphonage. The bag should either be pinned to the side of the bed or supported on a metal frame. It should not be allowed to lie on the floor. The length of the drainage system should be appropriately long to avoid traction on the urethra. It should be remembered that, in the absence of obstruction, many UTIs will resolve when the catheter is removed. It is, therefore, not beneficial to treat all cases of bacteriuria. Antibiotics should be reserved for symptomatic patients since treatment will only allow the establishment of resistant bacteria. Bladder lavage can be useful in controlling symptoms in patients who are catheterized long term.

ILEAL LOOPS

It should come as no surprise that the ileal loop becomes colonized with its own flora. Usually, one particular strain predominates and it can become very difficult to eradicate. *Pseudomonas* species, once established, can rarely be dislodged. Various approaches to colonization may be tried. It is important that the loop is fashioned correctly. If the urine is traversing it in an antiperistaltic manner, hydronephrosis and ascending infection will result. The length of the loop must be calculated carefully. Too long a loop will result in pooling of urine. This will predispose to increased colonization. Stoma appliances should be changed regularly since they are almost impossible to keep acceptably free from significant levels of bacteria. The stoma nurse has much to contribute to the management of these patients and can advise about positioning the stoma preoperatively. Regular support is valuable, not only to boost morale but in managing leaks.

Woodhouse and his colleagues[22] reviewed the long-term results of patients who had a uretero-sigmoid diversion for a mean period of 20 years. About half had hyperchloraemic acidosis but there was an appreciable risk of benign and malignant neoplasia. This requires at least annual colonoscopy. It is thought that the risk of malignancy is related to carriage of *Peptostreptococcus* species. The high level of upper urinary tract sepsis has, however, discouraged this approach and many urologists convert patients with a utero-sigmoid diversion to a stoma.

There has been a trend recently to reverse previous diversionary procedures, and this step may procure reasonable urinary control and reduce sepsis. The decision to re-operate should be taken only after detailed pressure studies have been analysed.

ANTIBIOTIC PROPHYLAXIS FOR UROLOGICAL OPERATIONS

Prophylactic antibiotics should be used with two principles in mind. First, that the chosen antibiotic should be effective against the likely pathogens, and, second, that it is given to achieve high tissue levels at the time of surgery without provoking toxicity or the emergence of resistant strains.

The incidence of bacteraemia and septicaemia after urological procedures is shown to be high and is well documented[23,24]. Guidelines have been proposed[25,26] for prophylactic antibiotics in urological surgery but a survey of urological surgeons in Britain in 1985[27] showed that a standard format had not been achieved. At present, because of the high risk of postoperative sepsis, peroperative antibiotics are routinely used for percutaneous nephrolithotomy (PCN). This is particularly necessary when the stone is a staghorn. We do not know if, in the long term, the incidence of urinary tract infection will be reduced. Opinions are divided as to the necessity for prophylactic antibiotics after routine surgery and perhaps they are only required in high-risk patients, such as diabetic and immunocompromised patients. Where there has been an indwelling catheter, antibiotics are a wise precaution. Spinal injury patients have a high risk of sepsis and most surgeons would employ appropriate prophylaxis in this group.

REFERENCES

1. Scott, J. E. S. (1987). Ureteric reflux: the present position. In Hendry, W. F. (ed.) *Recent Advances in Urology/Andrology*, No. **4**, pp. 89–108. (Edinburgh: Churchill Livingstone)
2. O'Donnell, B. and Puri, P. (1984). Treatment of vesicoureteric reflux by endoscopic injection of Teflon. *Br. Med. J.,* **289,** 7–9
3. Norden, C. W. and Kass, E. H. (1968). Bacteriuria of pregnancy – A critical appraisal. *Ann. Rev. Med.,* **19,** 431–470
4. Sweet, R. L. (1977). Bacteriuria and pyelonephritis during pregnancy. *Semin. Perinatol.,* **1,** 25–40
5. Kreiger, J. N. (1986). Complications and treatment of urinary tract infections during pregnancy. *Urol. Clin. N. Am.,* **13** (4), 685–693
6. File Jr., T. M. and Tan, J. S. (1986). Empiric antimicrobial therapy of serious urinary tract infections. *Urology,* **27,** 80–85
7. Roberts, J. A. (1986) Pyelonephritis, cortical abscess and perinephric abscess. *Urol. Clin. N. Am.,* **13** (4), 637–645

8. Lim, F. T. K. S. (1985). Sexually transmitted diseases. In Whitfield, H. N. and Hendry, W. F. (eds.) *Textbook of Genito-Urinary Surgery,* Vol. 1, pp. 579–586. (Edinburgh: Churchill Livingstone)

9. Willox, R. R. (1981. International trends affecting the control of the sexually transmitted diseases. In Harris, J. R. W. (ed.) *Recent Advances in S.T.D.,* No. 2, pp. 1–34. (Edinburgh: Churchill Livingstone)

10. Gellan, M. C. A. and Ison, C. A. (1986). Declining incidence of gonorrhoea in London: a response to fear of AIDS? *Lancet,* **2,** 920–922

11. Kenn, C. and Goorney, B. (1988). Changes in sexual attitudes and behaviour in the light of increased awareness of AIDS. *Br. J. Sex. Med.,* **15,** 162–165

12. Cinman, A, C. (1982). Tuberculosis. *Urology,* **20,** 353–358

13. Gow J. G. (1986). Genitourinary tuberculosis. In Walsh, P. C., Gittes, R. F., Perlmutter, A. D. and Stamey, T. A. (eds.) *Campbells Urology,* 5th Edn, Vol. 1, pp. 1037–1061. (Philadelphia: Saunders)

14. Fox, W. (1981). Whither short course chemotherapy? *Br. J. Dis. Chest,* **75,** 331–357

15. Gow, J. G. and Barbosa, S. (1984). Genitourinary tuberculosis. A study of 1117 cases over a period of 34 years. *Br. J. Urol.,* **56,** 449–455

16. McAllister, W. A. C., Thompson, P. J., Al-Habet, S. M. and Rogers, H. J. (1983). Rifampicin reduces effectiveness and bioavailability of prednisolone. *Br. Med. J.,* **286,** 923–925

17. Dounis, A., Abel, B. J. and Gow, J. G. (1980). Caecocystoplasty for bladder augmentation. *J. Urol.,* **123,** 164–167

18. Drach, G. W. and Nolan, J. P. E. (1986). Chronic bacterial prostatitis: Problems in diagnosis and therapy. *Urology,* **27** (suppl), 26–30

19. Meares, E. M. Jr (1982). Prostatitis: review of pharmacokinetics and therapy. *Rev. Infect. Dis.,* **4,** 475–483

20. Fowler, J. E. Jr and Marshall, V. (1983). Nosocomial catheter-associated urinary tract infections. *Infect. Surg.,* **2,** 43–47

21. Garibaldi, R. A., Burke, J. P., Dickman, M. L. and Smith, C. B. (1974). Factors predisposing to bacteriuria during indwelling urethral catherization. *N. Engl. J. Med.,* **291,** 215–219

22. Silverman, S. H., Woodhouse, C. R. J., Strachan, J. R., Cumming, J. and Keighley, M. R. B. (1986). Longterm management of patients who have had urinary diversions into colon. *Br. J. Urol.,* **58,** 634–639

23. Robinson, M. R. G., Cross, R. J., Shetty, M. B. and Fitall, B. (1980). Bacteraemia and bacteriogenic shock in district hospital urological practice. *Br. J. Urol.,* **52,** 10–14

24. Sim, A. J. W. and McCartney, A. C. (1980). Endotoxaemia following urethral instrumentation. *Br. J. Surg.,* **67,** 443–445

25. Chisholm, G. D. (1982). Antimicrobial prophylaxis in urology and transplantation. *World J. Surg.,* **6,** 281–292

26. Russo, P., Packer, M. G. and Fair, W. G. (1983). Prophylactic antibiotics in urological surgery. *Semin. Urol.,* **1,** 155–163

27. Wilson, N. I. L. and Lewi, H. J. E. (1985). Survey of antibiotic prophylaxis in British urological practice. *Br. J. Urol.,* **57,** 478–482

INDEX